MW01079427

Roger N. Reeb
Editor

Community Action Research: Benefits to Community Members and Service Providers

Community Action Research: Benefits to Community Members and Service Providers has been co-published simultaneously as *Journal of Prevention & Intervention in the Community*, Volume 32, Numbers 1/2 2006.

"COMMUNITY MEMBERS WILL BENEFIT from a volume that presents a broad range of community service projects that have been evaluated. Exposure such as this may stimulate communities to develop their own action projects. RESEARCHERS WILL BENEFIT from the wide range of community projects that are described, and gain insight on how to evaluate these projects, from using qualitative approaches to standardized self-report measures that assess constructs specific to community action. In summary, individuals interested in developing community action projects and researchers interested in evaluating community service projects will find much USEFUL INFORMATION in this volume."

Anthony Spirito, PhD, ABPP
Professor of Psychiatry
and Human Behavior
Brown Medical School

"This VERY READABLE AND INTERESTING volume addresses a number of important and neglected topics in applied community psychology. Of particular value is its emphasis on the implementation of research in application to emergent community-level concerns. These include diversion alternatives for adolescents in juvenile courts, substance abuse in indigenous populations, neighborhood activism and community service, elder care, literacy, and service-learning programs for health professionals and educators. This emphasis on implementation bridges a gap that too often separates researchers and theoreticians from workers actually involved in working with community problems. Another notable strength of Reeb's book also involves the integration of scholarly efforts that are too often separate, in its use of quantitative as well as qualitative data. Several chapters also contribute to a pervasive multicultural perspective, including consideration of Alaskan natives, geoculturally distinct communities in Tasmania, and inner-city minority Philadelphia youth. Rigorous psychometric evaluation of assessment instruments needed in community research are presented along with a variety of intervention approaches. This fine book is CERTAIN TO BE OF CONSIDERABLE VALUE to students, researchers and practitioners in community psychology, and in particular to those concerned with the integration of research and practice in this important area."

Joseph P. Bush, PhD
Associate Dean and Faculty
School of Psychology
Fielding Graduate University

Community Action Research:
Benefits to Community Members
and Service Providers

Community Action Research: Benefits to Community Members and Service Providers has been co-published simultaneously as *Journal of Prevention & Intervention in the Community*, Volume 32, Numbers 1/2 2006.

Journal of Prevention & Intervention in the Community is the successor title to *Prevention in Human Services*, which changed title after Vol. 12, No. 2 1995. *Journal of Prevention & Intervention in the Community*, under its new title, began with Volume 13, No. 1/2 1996.

Traumatic Stress and Its Aftermath: Cultural, Community, and Professional Contexts, edited by Sandra S. Lee, PhD (Vol. 26, No. 1, 2003). *Explores risk and protective factors for traumatic stress, emphasizing the impact of cumulative/multiple trauma in a variety of populations, including therapists themselves.*

Culture, Peers, and Delinquency, edited by Clifford O'Donnell, PhD (Vol. 25, No. 2, 2003). *"Timely . . . . of value to both students and professionals. . . . Demonstrates how peers can serve as a pathway to delinquency from a multiethnic perspective. The discussion of ethnic, racial, and gender differences challenges the field to reconsider assessment, treatment, and preventative approaches." (Donald Meichenbaum, PhD, Distinguished Professor Emeritus, University of Waterloo, Ontario, Canada; Research Director, The Melissa Institute for Violence Prevention and the Treatment of Victims of Violence, Miami, Florida)*

Prevention and Intervention Practice in Post-Apartheid South Africa, edited by Vijé Franchi, PhD, and Norman Duncan, PhD, consulting editor (Vol. 25, No.1, 2003). *"Highlights the way in which preventive and curative interventions serve–or do not serve–the ideals of equality, empowerment, and participation. . . . Revolutionizes our way of thinking about and teaching socio-pedagogical action in the context of exclusion." (Dr. Altay A. Manço, Scientific Director, Institute of Research, Training, and Action on Migrations, Belgium)*

Community Interventions to Create Change in Children, edited by Lorna H. London, PhD (Vol. 24, No. 2, 2002). *"Illustrates creative approaches to prevention and intervention with at-risk youth . . . . Describes multiple methods to consider in the design, implementation, and evaluation of programs." (Susan D. McMahon, PhD, Assistant Professor, Department of Psychology, DePaul University)*

Preventing Youth Access to Tobacco, edited by Leonard A. Jason, PhD, and Steven B. Pokorny, PhD (Vol. 24, No. 1, 2002). *"Explores cutting-edge issues in youth access research methodology. . . . Provides a thorough review of the tobacco control literature and detailed analysis of the methodological issues presented by community interventions to increase the effectiveness of tobacco control. . . . Challenges widespread assumptions about the dynamics of youth access programs and the requirements for long-term success." (John A. Gardiner, PhD, LLB, Consultant to the 2000 Surgeon General's Report* Reducing Youth Access to Tobacco *and to the National Cancer Institute's evaluation of the ASSIST program)*

The Transition from Welfare to Work: Processes, Challenges, and Outcomes, edited by Sharon Telleen, PhD, and Judith V. Sayad (Vol. 23, No. 1/2, 2002). *A comprehensive examination of the welfare-to-work initiatives surrounding the major reform of United States welfare legislation in 1996.*

Prevention Issues for Women's Health in the New Millennium, edited by Wendee M. Wechsberg, PhD (Vol. 22, No. 2, 2001). *"Helpful to service providers as well as researchers . . . A Useful ancillary textbook for courses addressing women's health issues. Covers a wide range of health issues affecting women." (Sherry Deren, PhD, Director, Center for Drug Use and HIV Research, National Drug Research Institute, New York City)*

Workplace Safety: Individual Differences in Behavior, edited by Alice F. Stuhlmacher, PhD, and Douglas F. Cellar, PhD (Vol. 22, No. 1, 2001). Workplace Safety: Individual Differences in Behavior *examines safety behavior and outlines practical interventions to help increase safety awareness. Individual differences are relevant to a variety of settings, including the workplace, public spaces, and motor vehicles. This book takes a look at ways of defining and measuring safety as well as a variety of individual differences like gender, job knowledge, conscientiousness, self-efficacy, risk avoidance, and stress tolerance that are important in creating safety interventions and improving the selection and training of employees.* Workplace Safety *takes an incisive look at these issues with a unique focus on the way individual differences in people impact safety behavior in the real world.*

People with Disabilities: Empowerment and Community Action, edited by Christopher B. Keys, PhD, and Peter W. Dowrick, PhD (Vol. 21, No. 2, 2001). *"Timely and useful . . . provides valuable lessons and guidance for everyone involved in the disability movement. This book is a must-read for researchers and practitioners interested in disability rights issues!" (Karen M. Ward, EdD, Director, Center for Human Development; Associate Professor, University of Alaska, Anchorage)*

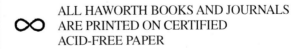

Community Action Research:
Benefits to Community Members
and Service Providers

Roger N. Reeb
Editor

Community Action Research: Benefits to Community Members and Service Providers has been co-published simultaneously as *Journal of Prevention & Intervention in the Community*, Volume 32, Numbers 1/2 2006.

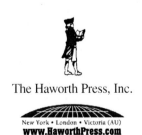

The Haworth Press, Inc.

New York • London • Victoria (AU)
www.HaworthPress.com

Community Action Research: Benefits to Community Members and Service Providers has been co-published simultaneously as *Journal of Prevention & Intervention in the Community*, Volume 32, Numbers 1/2 2006.

The development, preparation, and publication of this work has been undertaken with great care. However, the publisher, employees, editors, and agents of The Haworth Press and all imprints of The Haworth Press, Inc., including The Haworth Medical Press® and Pharmaceutical Products Press®, are not responsible for any errors contained herein or for consequences that may ensue from use of materials or information contained in this work. With regard to case studies, identities and circumstances of individuals discussed herein have been changed to protect confidentiality. Any resemblance to actual persons, living or dead, is entirely coincidental.

The Haworth Press is committed to the dissemination of ideas and information according to the highest standards of intellectual freedom and the free exchange of ideas. Statements made and opinions expressed in this publication do not necessarily reflect the views of the Publisher, Directors, management, or staff of The Haworth Press, Inc., or an endorsement by them.

Cover design by Kerry E. Mack

Library of Congress Cataloging-in-Publication Data

Community action research: benefits to community members and service providers / Roger N. Reeb, editor.
     p. cm.
    "Co-published simultaneously as Journal of prevention & intervention in the community, volume 32, numbers 1/2 2006."
    Includes bibliographical references and index.
    ISBN-13: 978-0-7890-3046-7 (hard cover : alk. paper)
    ISBN-10: 0-7890-3046-2 (hard cover : alk. paper)
    ISBN-13: 978-0-7890-3047-4 (soft cover : alk. paper)
    ISBN-10: 0-7890-3047-0 (soft cover : alk. paper)
    1. Paraprofessionals in social service–Research. 2. Volunteer workers in social service–Research. 3. Community psychology–Research. 4. Action research. 5. Evaluation research (Social action programs) I. Reeb, Roger N. II. Journal of prevention & intervention in the community.
HV40.4.C65 2006
361.8–dc22

                                        2005018299

Indexing, Abstracting & Website/Internet Coverage

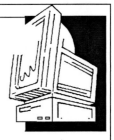

This section provides you with a list of major indexing & abstracting services and other tools for bibliographic access. That is to say, each service began covering this periodical during the year noted in the right column. Most Websites which are listed below have indicated that they will either post, disseminate, compile, archive, cite or alert their own Website users with research-based content from this work. (This list is as current as the copyright date of this publication.)

Abstracting, Website/Indexing Coverage . . . . Year When Coverage Began

- *(IBZ) International Bibliography of Periodical Literature on the Humanities and Social Sciences (Thomson)* <http://www.saur.de> 1997

- *Behavioral Medicine Abstracts* 1996

- *Cambridge Scientific Abstracts is a leading publisher of scientific information in print journals, online databases, CD-ROM and via the Internet <http://www.csa.com>* 2006

- *CINAHL (Cumulative Index to Nursing & Allied Health Literature) (EBSCO) <http://www.cinahl.com>* 2003

- *EBSCOhost Electronic Journals Service (EJS)* <http://ejournals.ebsco.com> 2001

- *Educational Research Abstracts (ERA) (online database)* <http://www.tandf.co.uk/era> 2002

- *Elsevier Scopus <http://www.info.scopus.com>* 2005

- *EMBASE.com (The Power of EMBASE + MEDLINE Combined) <http://www.embase.com>* . . . . *

- *EMBASE/Excerpta Medica Secondary Publishing Division. Included in newsletters, review journals, major reference works, magazines & abstract journals <http://www.elsevier.nl>* 1996

- *Excerpta Medica . . . See EMBASE* . . . . *

(continued)

(continued)

- *Social Work Abstracts*
  <http://www.silverplatter.com/catalog/swab.htm> **1996**
- *SocIndex (EBSCO)* **2003**
- *Sociological Abstracts (Cambridge Scientific Abstracts)*
  <http://www.csa.com> **1998**
- *SwetsWise <http://www.swets.com>* **2001**
- *Violence and·Abuse Abstracts: A Review of Current*
  Literature on Interpersonal Violence (VAA). **1996**
- *Women, Girls & Criminal Justice Newsletter* **2004**

*Exact start date to come.

Special Bibliographic Notes related to special journal issues
(separates) and indexing/abstracting:

- indexing/abstracting services in this list will also cover material in any "separate" that is co-published simultaneously with Haworth's special thematic journal issue or DocuSerial. Indexing/abstracting usually covers material at the article/chapter level.
- monographic co-editions are intended for either non-subscribers or libraries which intend to purchase a second copy for their circulating collections.
- monographic co-editions are reported to all jobbers/wholesalers/approval plans. The source journal is listed as the "series" to assist the prevention of duplicate purchasing in the same manner utilized for books-in-series.
- to facilitate user/access services all indexing/abstracting services are encouraged to utilize the co-indexing entry note indicated at the bottom of the first page of each article/chapter/contribution.
- this is intended to assist a library user of any reference tool (whether print, electronic, online, or CD-ROM) to locate the monographic version if the library has purchased this version but not a subscription to the source journal.
- individual articles/chapters in any Haworth publication are also available through the Haworth Document Delivery Service (HDDS).

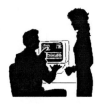

Community Action Research: Benefits to Community Members and Service Providers

CONTENTS

ABOUT THE EDITOR

Roger N. Reeb, PhD, is Associate Professor of Psychology in the Department of Psychology at the University of Dayton, Ohio, Dr. Reeb received his PhD in Clinical Psychology in 1993 from Virginia Commonwealth University, where he met requirements for child, adult, and health psychology tracks. After completing his pre-doctoral internship at Brown University Clinical Psychology Internship Consortium in 1993, Dr. Reeb joined the faculty at the University of Dayton. Dr. Reeb has received the following awards from the American Psychological Association: American Psychological Association Dissertation Award in 1991; and the Springer Award for Excellence in Research in Rehabilitation Psychology (Research Committee of Division 22 of the American Psychological Association) in 1994. At the University of Dayton, Dr. Reeb has received awards for his research and teaching in the area of service-learning (Outstanding Faculty Service-Learning Award in 1997 and the Service-Learning Faculty Research Award in 1998), and he was nominated for the National 1998 Campus Compact Thomas Ehrlich Faculty Award for Service-Learning. Dr. Reeb has developed several lines of research interests in the areas of health and pediatric psychology, stress and coping, self-efficacy theory, classification and assessment of psychopathology, eating disorders, and service-learning effectiveness. In addition, Dr. Reeb has published over 20 refereed articles and has made over 45 professional conference presentations.

Foreword

Discourse on community involvement during the past decade, including community-based research, has shifted models of community engagement from those in which experts disseminate information to communities or use the community as the object of their research to models that emphasize values and processes that encompass participatory collaboration (e.g., community representatives as co-researchers and co-educators), democratic processes, and honoring different ways of knowing. The focus of these new models is not on where the activity occurs (e.g., "in the community"), but how the activity occurs (e.g., "in and with the community"; Bringle, Hatcher, & Clayton, in press). Many have built upon Boyer's (1996) thinking and offered critical examinations of how new models for engagement may change the nature of faculty work, enhance student learning, better fulfill campus mission, influence strategic planning and assessment, and improve campus-community relations (e.g., Bringle, Games, & Malloy, 1999a; Calleson, Jordan, & Seifer, 2005; Colby, Ehrlich, Beaumont, & Stephens, 2003; Eggerton, 1994).

This volume fits the zeitgeist of the academic community furthering its understanding of *Community Action Research* among students and among adults in the community. These case studies illustrate, to varying degrees and in different ways, how research may be collaborative processes with communities to promote social change and benefit both community members and service providers. Researchers who undertake work that combines community involvement with scholarship (e.g., participatory research) discover enriched rewards for themselves and others. However, this work raises broader issues about the acad-

[Haworth indexing entry note]: "Foreword." Bringle, Robert G. *Community Action Research: Benefits to Community Members and Service Providers* (ed: Roger N. Reeb) The Haworth Press, Inc., 2006, pp. xv-xvi. Single or multiple copies of this article are available for a fee from The Haworth Document Delivery Service [1-800-HAWORTH, 9:00 a.m. - 5:00 p.m. (EST). E-mail address: docdelivery@haworthpress.com].

emy's capacity to honor and reward it. Thus, Walshok (1999) has proposed that each campus seriously consider the following questions:

- Are you asking faculty to account for the *public meaning and impact* of their scholarship beyond the discipline or profession?
- How is civic engagement presented as an *intellectual imperative*?
- How is the institution *intentionally* supporting faculty (e.g., enabling infrastructures) with an interest in civic engagement activities?

The future of *Community Action Research* will be influenced by the answers that each campus develops to these questions.

Robert G. Bringle, PhD
Chancellor's Professor of Psychology and Philanthropic Studies
Center for Service and Learning
Indiana University-Purdue University Indianapolis
June, 2006

REFERENCES

Boyer, E. L. (1996). The scholarship of engagement. *Journal of Public Service and Outreach, 1*, 11-20.

Bringle, R. G., Games, R., & Malloy, E. A. (1999a). *Colleges and universities as citizens*. Needham Heights, MA: Allyn and Bacon.

Bringle, R. G., Hatcher, J. A., & Clayton, P. (in press). The scholarship of civic engagement: Defining, documenting, and evaluating faculty work. *To Improve the Academy*.

Calleson, D. C., Jordan, C., & Seifer, S. D. (2005). Community-engaged scholarship: Is faculty work in communities a true academic enterprise? *Academic Medicine, 80*, 317-321.

Colby A., Ehrlich T., Beaumont E., & Stephens, J. (2003). *Educating citizens: Preparing America's undergraduates for lives of moral and civic responsibility*. San Francisco: Jossey-Bass. Eggerton, R. (1994). The engaged campus: Organizing to serve society's needs. *AAHE Bulletin, 47*, 2-3.

Eggerton, R. (1994). The engaged campus: Organizing to serve society's needs. *AAHE Bulletin, 47*, 2-3.

Walshok, M. L. (1999). Strategies for building the infrastructure that supports the engaged campus. In R.G. Bringle, R. Games, & E.A. Malloy (Eds.), *Colleges and universities as citizens* (pp. 74-95). Needham Heights, MA: Allyn & Bacon.

Community Action Research: An Introduction

Roger N. Reeb

University of Dayton

As community psychology developed, the utilization of paraprofessionals and volunteers in the provision of services proliferated (National Institute of Mental Health, 1970; Sobey, 1970). A *paraprofessional* is a worker who lacks an advanced degree but receives training and supervision by a professional so that he or she is able to perform certain tasks formerly performed by professional workers only. While paraprofessionals are typically paid for their services, *volunteers* actively engage in the provision of services due to other motivational factors (Clary, Snyder, Ridge, Copeland, Stukas, Haugen, & Miene, 1998), such as: an altruistic or humanitarian concern for one's community; a desire for opportunities for new learning experiences; social needs (affiliation or recognition); a wish to explore or clarify career options; a need to avoid or escape personal problems (e.g., guilt, loneliness); or self-esteem enhancement.

A culture-related gap exists between middle-class professionals and individuals from lower socioeconomic backgrounds who need services. When paraprofessionals and volunteers have socioeconomic backgrounds similar to community members receiving services, this helps to bridge the culture-related gap. Further, the utilization of volunteers and paraprofessionals has functioned to expand the base of personnel available to de-

[Haworth co-indexing entry note]: "Community Action Research: An Introduction." Reeb, Roger N. Co-published simultaneously in *Journal of Prevention & Intervention in the Community* (The Haworth Press, Inc.) Vol. 32, No. 1/2, 2006, pp. 1-4; and: *Community Action Research: Benefits to Community Members and Service Providers* (ed: Roger N. Reeb) The Haworth Press, Inc., 2006, pp. 1-4. Single or multiple copies of this article are available for a fee from The Haworth Document Delivery Service [1-800-HAWORTH, 9:00 a.m. - 5:00 p.m. (EST). E-mail address: docdelivery@haworthpress.com].

liver services (NIMH, 1970; Sobey, 1970). As delineated below, the articles in the special volume provide samples of research in two general lines of investigation in community psychology that have developed due to the increasingly common utilization of paraprofessionals and volunteers in service provision.

One goal of community psychology is to apply psychological theory and research in ways that enhance the *psychological wellness* of community members (Cowan, 1991, 1994). As community psychology was developing a distinctive identity, it became evident that community programs utilizing paraprofessionals and volunteers were beneficial to community members (Alley, Blanton, Feldman, Hunter, & Rolfson, 1979). The first section of this special volume, *Community Action Research: Benefits to Community Members*, presents a sample of studies that (a) utilized volunteers or paraprofessionals in the implementation of services or social action, and (b) demonstrated benefits of the program to members of the community.

In the first section, Sturza and Davidson report results of their research on the Adolescent Diversion Project, which is an intervention strategy that utilizes volunteers and students as change agents and serves as an alternative to juvenile court. Oneal, Reeb, Korte, and Butter examine the reliability and validity of a psychometric instrument that was designed to be used by paraprofessionals to monitor changes in the symptoms of autistic youngsters over the course of home-based behavior modification. Allen, Mohatt, Rasmus, Hazel, Thomas, Lindley, and the People Awakening Project Team present the results of research in which paraprofessionals played a major role in the identification of protective factors in Alaska Native sobriety and the designing of a preventative intervention. Donnelly and Kimble examine the outcomes of a crime prevention project implemented by a residential neighborhood association. Dowrick and Yuen review the effects of the ACE (Actual Community Empowerment) Reading Program, which utilized community members as literacy tutors.

Constructs examined in community psychology, such as empowerment, psychological empowerment, citizen participation, social justice, competence (and self-efficacy), and sense of community (see Rappaport & Seidman, 2000), are central to understanding (a) why some individuals pursue volunteerism and/or paraprofessional work, as well as (b) changes in personal development that take place in individuals as a consequence of community service involvement. The second section of this special volume, *Community Action Research, Benefits to Service Providers*, presents studies that demonstrate benefits in personal development for volunteers and paraprofessionals providing services in community members.

In the second section, Reeb provides further evidence of reliability and validity for the Community Service Self-Efficacy Scale, which is a psychometric instrument designed to assess " . . . the individual's confidence in his or her own ability to make clinically significant contributions to the community though service." Ferrari, Kapoor, Bristow, and Woods Bowman examine community service self-efficacy, psychological sense of community, and emotional experiences of caregivers for the elderly in Tasmania, Australia. Olney, Livingston, Fisch, and Talamantes examine the learning and socio-emotional outcomes for medical students in a community service-learning project. Yamauchi, Billig, Meyer, and Hofschire examine improvements in the sense of community and other beneficial outcomes for students participating in the Hawaiian Studies Program, which involves weekly participation in community service-learning exercises.

The articles presented in this special volume advance our understanding of the potential benefits of research that utilize volunteers or paraprofessionals as change agents. It is hoped that these articles stimulate further research examining the benefits of community-based research projects for both (a) members of the community in need of services, and (b) volunteers and paraprofessionals providing community service.

REFERENCES

Alley, S., Blanton, J., Feldman, R. E., Hunter, G. D., & Rolfson, M. (1979). *Case studies of mental health paraprofessionals. Twelve effective programs.* New York: Human Sciences Press.

Clary, E. G., Snyder, M., Ridge, R. D., Copeland, J., Stukas, A. A., Haugen, J., & Miene, P. (1998). Understanding and assessing the motivations of volunteers: A functional analysis. *Journal of Personality and Social Psychology, 74,* 1516-1530.

Cowan, E. L. (1991). In pursuit of wellness. *American Psychologist, 46,* 404-408.

Cowan, E. L. (1994). The enhancement of psychological wellness: Challenges and opportunities. *American Journal of Community Psychology, 22,* 149-180.

National Institute of Mental Health (1970). *Volunteers in community mental health.* Washington, DC: U.S. Government Printing Office.

Rappaport, J., & Seidman, E. (Eds.). (2000). *Handbook of community psychology.* New York: Kluwer Academic/Plenum Publishers.

Sobey, F. (1970). *The nonprofessional revolution in mental health.* New York: Columbia University Press.

PART I:
COMMUNITY ACTION RESEARCH:
BENEFITS TO COMMUNITY MEMBERS

Issues Facing the Dissemination of Prevention Programs: Three Decades of Research on the Adolescent Diversion Project

Marisa L. Sturza
William S. Davidson II

Michigan State University

Marisa L. Sturza is a Doctoral Candidate, at Michigan State University, Department of Psychology, 135 Snyder Hall, MSU, E. Lansing, MI 48824-1117 (E-mail: sturzama@msu.edu).

William S. Davidson II is University Distinguished Professor, Chair, Ecological-Community Psychology Graduate Program, and Editor, *American Journal of Community Psychology*, Michigan State University, Department of Psychology 135 Snyder Hall, MSU, E. Lansing, MI 48824-1117 (E-mail: davidso7@msu.edu).

[Haworth co-indexing entry note]: "Issues Facing the Dissemination of Prevention Programs: Three Decades of Research on the Adolescent Diversion Project." Sturza, Marisa L. and William S. Davidson II. Co-published simultaneously in *Journal of Prevention & Intervention in the Community* (The Haworth Press, Inc.) Vol. 32, No. 1/2, 2006, pp. 5-24; and: *Community Action Research: Benefits to Community Members and Service Providers* (ed: Roger N. Reeb) The Haworth Press, Inc., 2006, pp. 5-24. Single or multiple copies of this article are available for a fee from The Haworth Document Delivery Service [1-800-HAWORTH, 9:00 a.m. - 5:00 p.m. (EST). E-mail address: docdelivery@haworthpress.com].

SUMMARY. This paper argues that the issues facing effective prevention programs when they embark on dissemination, implementation, and routinization have been largely ignored by the field. Through the example of the Adolescent Diversion Program, these issues are illustrated and discussed. Four sequential longitudinal experimental studies are summarized as a context for the discussion of dissemination issues. In each case, the alternative preventive program is demonstrated to be more effective than traditional approaches. Challenges to widespread implementation of effective prevention programs are then discussed with a call for the field to add such issues to its scientific agenda. *[Article copies available for a fee from The Haworth Document Delivery Service: 1-800-HAWORTH. E-mail address: <docdelivery@haworthpress.com> Website: <http://www.HaworthPress.com> © 2006 by The Haworth Press, Inc. All rights reserved.]*

KEYWORDS. Prevention, prevention program, juvenile delinquency treatment, dissemination

After nearly 30 years of operation, the Adolescent Diversion Project (ADP) has continued to divert youth from traditional juvenile court processing as a method of preventing future delinquency. The program has been focused on intervention methods which create an alternative to juvenile court within a strengths-based, advocacy framework (e.g., Davidson et al., 1990). In multiple randomized trials, ADP has demonstrated that youth exposed to alternative preventive interventions have lower rates of recidivism compared to youth who have either undergone traditional juvenile court processing or been released without further intervention. Further, the ADP costs a fraction of what traditional court processing does (Davidson et al., 1990; Davidson et al., 2000, Davidson & Redner, 1988; Smith et al., 2004). Also, the ADP has found that youth participating in the program have exhibited increased involvement with families, schools, employment, and reported overall positive experiences with the intervention (Davidson et al., 1990; Davidson et al., 2000). In addition, ADP has demonstrated that students working as advocates have reported increased political commitment (Angelique, 2002). For the purposes of the present paper, the outcomes of reduced recidivism rates and cost will be focused on. The present paper will provide a description of the history of the ADP, a summary of prior research on the program, and outline challenges facing effective alternative prevention models as they seek adoption and routinization.

HISTORY OF THE ADOLESCENT DIVERSION PROJECT (ADP)

Research on the ADP model was first conducted in the 1970s and replicated/extended through the 1980s and 1990s (Davidson et al., 1977; Davidson et al., 2000; Smith et al., 2003). The original prototype continues to operate in partnership with a local county in order to provide prevention services for over 100 youth per year. Diverting youth from traditional juvenile court services is the foundation of ADP. This notion of youth diversion originated out of the President's 1967 Commission on Law Enforcement and Administration of Justice. This commission argued that the traditional system was so ineffective that alternatives had to be considered (Davidson et al., 2000; Gensheimer et al., 1986; President's Commission, 1967). The historical context for the development of the ADP model is important to understand. At the time of its inception, juvenile delinquency was a national priority. Further, it had been argued that the juvenile justice system was expensive, inhumane, and ineffective (Krisberg & Austin, 1976). It had even been argued that the traditional court increased future delinquency (e.g., Gold, 1974).

COMPONENTS OF ADP

Given the zeitgeist present at the time ADP was developed, it was clear that an alternative was needed. What was less clear was what should be done as an alternative. In other words, it was clear what not to do; it was less clear what to do. There were several prominent areas of research which were key to the original development of the ADP prevention model. First, as mentioned above, the creation of an alternative to the justice system (which became known as diversion) was recommended. Formally, the tenets of symbolic interactionism and labeling theory were central to design of the model. Second, the goal of providing preventive interventions which would minimize the negative effects of labeling and enhance positive expectations was included (e.g., Gold, 1974; Becker, 1968). The direct implication was that preventive interventions would best take place outside the formal court system and that the content of intervention should be positive in its focus. Third, at the time, a literature was beginning to develop which demonstrated that relatively intense interventions were more likely to be effective (Davidson et al., 1989; Lipsey, 1992). Finally, alternative preventive interventions (as is almost always the case) were expected to cost less.

Each of these factors played a key role in the development of the ADP model. The original preventive model occurred outside the juvenile justice system, accepting referrals from the juvenile division of a local police department as an alterative to formal prosecution. This structure had two advantages. First, it avoided the potential risks of overidentifying "potential delinquents" or "pre-delinquents" and ensured that the youth involved were truly at risk of official delinquency. Avoiding net widening was an important consideration (Sheldon, 1999). Second, it insured that the preventive intervention was truly an alternative to the formal system and hence preventive in its focus. This can be thought of as the systems level characteristics of this preventive program. Additionally, the preventive model involved individual-level intervention activities which were specific, positive, and intense. Originally, the promising alternatives of behavioral approaches (e.g., Patterson, 1971) and child advocacy (e.g., Davidson & Rapp, 1976) formed the basis of the individual-level intervention which took place in the diversion context. While relatively new on the scene of delinquency intervention at that juncture, both approaches had demonstrated considerable empirical promise (e.g., Davidson & Seidman, 1976), provided specific prescriptions for forming a preventive intervention model, and were strengths-based in their focus.

Finally, the intensity and cost of the preventive intervention had to be addressed. A related set of events was important in the construction of the ADP model. At the time, the systematic use of alternative person power groups (e.g., Rappaport et al., 1971) was achieving considerable promise. Further, the use of such groups as students and/or volunteers as change agents had demonstrated promising results while providing an inexpensive alternative for providing intense services (e.g., Tharp & Wetzel, 1969). Within this historical and theoretical context, the ADP prevention model was created. It involved the use of trained college students as change agents using behavioral and advocacy approaches in intense one-on-one preventive interventions in a diversionary, alternative context.

The major purpose of this article is to articulate the challenges successful prevention programs will face as they move from demonstrating their efficacy towards adoption as usual practice. To date, the preponderance of research on prevention has been focused on demonstrating efficacy. It has often been assumed that if effective alternatives are developed and demonstrated, widespread adoption will follow and routinization will follow (e.g., Mayer & Davidson, 2000). It is now clear that this is not the case, particularly as preventive alternatives are truly alternative and effective. The balance of this article will begin to elucidate the issues involved in these issues using the case of the ADP as an example. In order to set the stage for this discussion, the empirical history of ADP will be briefly reviewed for the reader not familiar with this empirical history. A relatively brief description of the outcome results of the ADP will be included here. For the interested reader, past studies presenting the results of the ADP over the past 25 to 30 years are provided in the Appendix.

OUTCOME RESEARCH ON THE ADP PREVENTION MODEL

Research evaluations of the ADP project have been broken up into four distinct phases (Davidson & Redner, 1988; Davidson et al., 1987; Smith et al., 2003). The purpose of the multi-phased project development has been to demonstrate reduced recidivism rates (Phase 1), determine the integrity and relative efficacy of the intervention components (Phase 2), examine the relative effectiveness of the types of advocates (Phase 3), and replicate the model in an urban setting allowing direct comparison of the model to usual processing (treatment as usual control) and outright release (no treatment control) (Phase 4).

Phase 1

In Phase 1, 73 youths participated, 84% who were male and 67% who were Caucasian. The conditions were dichotomized into treatment (ADP preventive intervention) and control (diversion without services). Preventive interventions were delivered one-on-one by college students (8 hours of intervention in the youth's environment per week), who were trained (80 hours of training) and supervised (two hours per week of supervision) in the use of behavioral contracting and child advocacy. The ADP group demonstrated significantly reduced recidivism rates when compared with the control group at both one and two-year follow-ups (Davidson et al,. 1977). While these results lent support to the ADP model of behavior contracting and advocacy, this was a preliminary study. The number of participants was relatively small and only a single city was involved. The need for systematic replication seemed paramount (see Table 1).

TABLE 1. Phase 1 Two-Year Follow-Up Recidivism Occurrences

Condition	n	Did not have further court contact	Had at least one additional contact with court
Behavioral Contracting/Advocacy	49	27	22
Control	24	1	23

Note. χ^2 = 17.68, df = 1; p < .001

Phase 2

Phase 2 built upon the treatment versus control design of Phase 1, but instead expanded the number and type of conditions in order to more specifically test the effects of the preventive intervention components. In Phase 2, 228 youths participated. The participants were 83% male and 74% Caucasian. The youths were randomly assigned to one of six conditions: Action (AC), Action Family-Focus (AC-FF), Action Court-Setting (AC-CS), Relationship (RC), Attention Placebo (APC), and Control (CC).

The Action, Action Family-Focus, and Action Court-Setting groups all involved advocacy and behavioral contracting. The difference between these three conditions was that the Action condition used behavioral contracting and advocacy to focus on all domains of the youth's life (e.g., family, school, peers, and employment), the Action Family-Focus used these techniques to focus exclusively on the youth's family, and the Action Court-Setting used these techniques within the context of court supervision. As a strategy to directly examine the effects of conducting preventive interventions outside the court system, student change agents in the Action Court-Setting group were trained by ADP staff, but supervised by juvenile court staff. In many ways, the Action Court-Setting group was the beginning of examining dissemination issues. Specifically, the question of what would happen to the efficacy of the preventive model when turned over to the existing system for operation was investigated.

The Relationship condition focused specifically on the relationship between the advocate and the youth without the advocacy and behavioral contracting components. The Relationship condition was a direct attempt to examine the impact of the relationship component of the preventive model. In other words, this phase explored what the effect would be of the relationship components of the intervention when they were evaluated in isolation.

The Attention Placebo condition did not have a structured model of intervention and was included in Phase 2 research to determine whether the Action conditions produced different outcomes than a nonspecific intervention. Finally, the Control condition was included to provide a treatment as usual control (Davidson et al., 1990).

Results from Phase 2 demonstrated that the only condition that significantly reduced recidivism when compared to the Attention Placebo group was the Action condition. The Action Family-Focus and Relationship groups were both superior to the treatment as usual control, but not more than the attention Placebo group. The Action Court-Setting group demonstrated the highest rate of recidivism, higher than the control (Davidson et al., 1990) (see Table 2).

Phase 3

After testing the relative efficacy of intervention components, Phase 3 sought to investigate whether the type of change agent was critical. University students had been enlisted in the previous two studies as advocates, but Phase 3 compared them to both community college students and general community volunteers. In Phase 3, 129 youths participated who were primarily male (83.9%) and Caucasian (70.2%). They were randomly assigned to university students, community college students, or community volunteers. Results from Phase 3 demonstrated that all groups were more effective than a treatment as usual control in

TABLE 2. Phase 2 Two-Year Cumulative Follow-Up Recidivism Occurrences

Condition	n	Did not have further court contact	Had at least one additional contact with court
Action	76	47	29
Action Family Focus	24	13	11
Action Court Setting	12	4	8
Relationship	12	8	4
Attention Placebo	29	14	15
Control	60	23	37

Note. $\chi^2 = 10.29$, df = 5; p < .07

reducing recidivism, indicating that the model was robust across type of change agent. The results also showed that the university students had more knowledge of the model, spent significantly more time with their youth, and the youth in this group reported having more positive experiences with their advocates. Evaluation of change agents in Phase 3 found that although there were significant benefits to using university students over the other two groups, community college students and community volunteers may also be effective advocates for this population (Davidson et al., 1990). In terms of recruitment, retention, and supervision, university students cost substantially less than the other two groups (see Table 3).

Phase 4

Phase 4 research examined three additional issues. First, it was important to replicate the preventive model beyond the medium-sized city populations of Phases 1 through 3. Second, it was important to examine the ADP model in comparison to treatment, as usual control as well as no treatment control within the same study. Third, it was important to see if the ADP model would be effective when implemented by paid professional staff. In Phase 4, the ADP model was implemented and tested in a large urban city (n = 395) with a population that was 84% male, and 90.6% African American. Youth were randomly assigned to either the ADP model, diversion without services (no treatment control), or traditional juvenile court processing (treatment as usual control). The urban replicate of ADP included both advocacy and behavior contracting components. The change agents in this phase were paid community members. At one year follow-up, the recidivism rates for

TABLE 3. Phase 3 Two-Year Cumulative Follow-Up Recidivism Occurrences

Condition	n	Did not have further court contact	Had at least one additional contact with court
University Student Advocates	47	30	17
Community College Student Advocates	35	26	9
Community Volunteer Advocates	17	13	4
Control	25	8	17

Note. $\chi^2 = 13.38$, df = 3; p < .01

youth who had completed the ADP model was significantly less than either the treatment as usual or no treatment controls (Davidson & Johnson, 1986; Smith et al., 2004) (see Table 4).

Phase 4 suggested that the ADP model could be effective with a youth population that is ethnically and geographically different from the population served in Phases 1 through 3 (Smith et al., 2004). Further, it demonstrated that ADP could be effective with community members as change agents.

Another important research finding from Phase 4 that has received less attention in the literature has been the lack of differential effects on youth who received traditional court services versus youth who received diversion without any services (Davidson et al., 1990; Davidson & Johnson, 1986; Smith et al., 2004). Diversion without services meant that youth were released with all charges dropped to return home to their parent(s)/guardian(s), with no further contact with the court system. In Phase 4, the recidivism rates for traditional court processing and diversion without services were nearly identical. This is interesting in that it replicates earlier work by Gold (1971) and Klein (1979) on which the diversion alternative was based. Phase 4 again calls into question the efficacy of usual court services. It is interesting to note that preventive alternatives are often held to the standard of demonstrating efficacy superior to traditional approaches when it may be that the typical approaches are themselves less than effective.

Further, Phase 4 demonstrated that the ADP prevention model produced superior recidivism rates in a random, longitudinal trial when compared to both youth who had received traditional juvenile court services and youth who had essentially received no intervention. Three additional studies, not discussed here and not involving the ADP prevention model, conducted in three different communities compared recidivism rates between youth randomly assigned to either traditional

TABLE 4. Phase 4 One-Year Follow-Up Recidivism Outcomes

Condition	n	Did not have further court contact	Had at least one additional contact with court
Family Support and Education	136	106	30
Diversion Without Services	135	92	43
Traditional Juvenile Court Processing	124	82	42

Note. $F = 40.13$, $df = 2$; $p < .001$

juvenile court processing or diversion without services. Each of these three studies found that the recidivism rates for these two groups of youth were not significantly different (Davidson & Johnson, 1986). Particularly important about these findings was that the three communities were unique from one another, including two mid-sized counties located in geographically distinct regions, and one small rural community.

Results in the first mid-sized county found that recidivism rates at one-year follow-up were identical for the traditional juvenile court processing group and the diversion without services group. Results in the second mid-sized county also found similar recidivism rates at one-year follow-up between youth in the juvenile court condition and youth in the diversion without services condition. Finally, in the rural community, rates were also similar for youth undergoing traditional court processing and for youth being diverted without services (Davidson & Johnson, 1986).

RELATIVE COST

In the collection of studies that evaluated three potential options– diversion with services, diversion without services, and traditional court processing–diversion without services was the most inexpensive option (Davidson & Johnson, 1986). Doing nothing typically costs the least in the short term. The most cost-effective services option was the ADP preventive model. The most costly option was traditional court processing (Davidson & Johnson, 1986).

Although the ADP prevention model has been demonstrated to be more inexpensive, there continues to be much larger proportions of money spent on traditional juvenile court services than on effective preventive alternatives. For example, in a recent analysis, ADP has cost approximately $1,020.83 per youth for an eighteen-week intervention, including all overhead and administrative costs. In comparison, the local juvenile court was spending $13,466 for the average youth served. While it must be noted that such comparisons are complex at best, these data derive from comparisons of expenditures on the same type of youth. Yet, these differences are rather striking. In a typical year, ADP provides preventive intervention to 144 youth, and the county juvenile court serves about 375 youth. The difference in cost of serving 144 youth in ADP versus traditional juvenile court results in a savings of approximately $1,799,104 per year.

DILEMMAS IN THE DISSEMINATION AND ROUTINIZATION OF EFFECTIVE PREVENTIVE ALTERNATIVES

The stage is now set for understanding the dissemination and routinization issues facing effective preventive programs. The ADP model has demonstrated its relative efficacy to traditional models of handling juvenile offenders, it has demonstrated that it is relatively cost effective, and it has demonstrated that traditional methods may be less than effective. This is precisely the situation described by scholars of dissemination. Current thinking in the dissemination of innovations provides a framework for this understanding. Various authors have described these processes as a dynamic and nonlinear set of stages. After demonstrating efficacy, an innovation is thought to go through stages of adoption, implementation, and routinization (Blakely et al., 1987; Mayer & Davidson, 2000).

In the adoption phase, the issue is whether the effective preventive intervention will be used by the relevant systems. Akin to the use of new pharmaceutical, the marketing metaphor has often been employed (Fairweather & Tornatzky, 1977; Mayer & Davidson, 2000). How to get the new preventive intervention to the stage of use is the question at hand.

In the implementation phase, the question becomes, "How will the intervention be carried out?" Will the original preventive intervention be used in a manner similar to the original so that fidelity occurs and similar outcomes can be assured? In the case of preventive interventions, the issues involve the inclusion of similar participants and the delivery of preventive interventions which mirror the original prototype.

In the routinization phase, the goal is that the preventive intervention becomes part of normal practice. Will the existing system use the more effective preventive intervention instead of prior, less effective practices? The goal of routinization is to have the more effective intervention be viewed as "the way we do things" rather than some new ancillary alternative.

As we begin to examine the applicability of this model to effective preventive interventions, as elucidated by our experience with the ADP model, a number of dilemmas arise. An often unstated assumption of alternative preventive interventions is that, if effective, they will reduce the incidence and prevalence of the social problem being addressed. If this is the case, then adoption should be expected. However, if successful, effective preventive interventions will result in less demand for and resulting use of traditional approaches. Yet, many preventive interventions are dependent upon the existing system for their source of participants (referrals) and even funding. In the case of the ADP preventive model, it is necessary for the existing juvenile justice system to refer youth to a traditional processing alternative. There are two potential outcomes of this which become problematic. First, if successful, the ADP model will reduce the demand for court services immediately by providing a dispositional alternative to court processing. In other words, youth diverted will not need a probation officer, court time, or residential treatment, etc. Second, if effective, future delinquency will be reduced, which will result in a further demand reduction for court services. This situation means that an existing system (in this case the juvenile justice system) will have to cooperate in adopting a program likely to ultimately reduce the size of that system. It seems that prevention programs, when successful, present a very clear-cut dilemma for the adoption phase of the process as currently conceived. In order to be adopted, effective preventive alternatives will need to compete for the very resources which support the status quo.

Another aspect of challenges to the prevailing paradigm occurs in the conceptualization of the implementation phase. Once adopted, it is important that an innovative prevention program operate in a manner congruent with the prototype which has been proven effective. In many cases, effective preventive interventions require role behaviors on the part of change agents which are incongruous with typical standard practice. For example, in the case of the ADP, it has been demonstrated important that innovative role behaviors including active case seeking, proactive intervention in the natural setting where youth live, high intensity of intervention, and positively oriented models of intervention are the likely sources of effectiveness. On the other hand, it is the typical practice for interventions within the juvenile justice system to be passive in their approach to case finding, "in the office" in their intervention modality, carrying caseloads where interventions are less than an hour per week, and following reactive, deterrence-based models of intervention. We know from the existing literature on implementation that high fidelity implementation is more likely to occur when the effective innovation requires performance patterns on the part of adoptees relatively congruent with current practice. The case in point is the example of the implementation of a new pharmaceutical for a known physical malady. High fidelity in such a situation requires a relatively small amount of change within an existing pattern of practice. Yet effective prevention programs, as in the case of the ADP, require major alterations in existing practice in order for true implementation to occur.

Further, Phase 2 research on the relative efficacy of the ADP indicated that routinization of prevention programs can also present challenges. Again, from the dissemination literature we know that routinization is an essential ingredient to long-term innovation stability. Becoming part of existing practice is the hallmark of innovation survival. Yet in the case of the ADP, the research indicated that turning over the preventive intervention to the existing justice system rather quickly destroyed its efficacy. However, it is at least an interesting observation that in order to become routinized, effective preventive programs may compromise their original impact.

To further elucidate these issues, the fiscal and organizational history of the ADP is instructive. Originally, the ADP was initiated with a large-scale federal grant from the National Institutes of Mental Health. With the use of "new outside" resources, adoption was accomplished. This is often the case during the development and demonstration of a new, effective preventive alternative. Our experience during these years was that adoption was relatively assured as long as external resources were available. Additionally, the independence of the effort (which Phase 2 research had demonstrated was critical) was easily maintained with outside funding.

After a decade and a half of external grant dollars, one variant of the ADP pursued continuation within the local funding situation. Since juvenile justice expenditures were a county-level responsibility in the state in question, the ADP proceeded to secure justice system support for continuation. Several amazing developments ensued. First, while the ADP had demonstrated its efficacy across four large-scale studies involving hundreds of youth, the local justice system, in budget hearings, argued that it simply could not afford to support the continuation of the ADP. Recall that the ADP model not only produced better outcomes, but did so at a fraction of the cost. To quote a judge, "I simply can't afford to lose a staff member to support this." The judge's view was that the budget required to support a more effective alternative translated into a loss of salary for an internal staff member. Second, the local legislative branch, foreseeing this challenge, chose to support continuation of the ADP, but outside the budget of the justice system. This had the dual effects of insuring the independence of the preventive alternative, yet at the same time presenting real challenges to routinization. Essentially, every year ADP funding was up for competition against other county departments. The need for political involvement in the dissemination process was magnified and the implied competition with the existing system was made public and explicit.

Specifically, the alternative, preventive nature of the ADP has created a significant barrier in its ability to move much further than the improvisation level of routinization. The ADP has displayed some of the characteristics of the improvisation level because of the long standing duration of the program, the weekly interaction it has with the juvenile court system, and its reliance on direct referrals by juvenile court officials to connect the youth population with the ADP. In fact, intakes of youth into the ADP are conducted by project staff at the county juvenile court. Further, funding for the project comes out of the same county fund as some of the services provided by the juvenile court. These are all examples of how the ADP has received some level of routinization into the juvenile court system.

On the contrary, there have also been examples demonstrating that the ADP has not achieved an expanded or disappearance level of routinization. First, the program has been considered a separate entity from the juvenile court by local government, the court, and the project itself. The juvenile court staff has not considered the ADP part of their domain. When it comes to budgeting, diversion has been considered separate from other juvenile court programs that come out of the same fund. Further, the project has considered itself affiliated with the university as opposed to the juvenile court. The question arises of whether it is possible for the program to become routinized into the court system while concurrently maintaining its founding ideology that it is a diversion from some of the negative effects that may result from involvement with juvenile court. Another example of how the ADP has not been considered a part of the court's daily activities is that the ADP has sometimes faced difficulties in receiving youth referrals from the court when compared with other youth programs that are internal, court-run programs. An additional struggle that has posed a challenge to the integration of the ADP has been the competition with the juvenile court for clients. The programs have not always been viewed as complementary, and the ADP has sometimes been viewed as a threat to the survival of the juvenile court programs. Both need youth to participate in order to function, yet there has been a limited pool of youth in the county who have been referred to juvenile court on a misdemeanor charge.

Also, another example of a barrier to the integration of the ADP has been the differences in values and theoretical orientations between the juvenile court and the ADP. The juvenile court has been operating on a treatment approach which believes that youth need to face the consequences of their actions, which is often enforced through punitive actions. Based on a different theoretical orientation, the ADP has aimed to work with youth as a form of secondary prevention. The ADP has selected youth who have committed misdemeanors and tried to intervene in order to prevent them from any further contact with the court system. The actual structure of the ADP has differed from the more punitive treatment of the juvenile court model in that it has tried to build upon the strengths of youth without including a punitive component. These theoretical differences between the court and the ADP may have also been a factor in preventing a higher level of routinization, closer to the expansion or disappearance levels. Clearly, although the ADP has been in the routinization stage of the dissemination of innovation model, there have been barriers preventing it from moving to a higher level within the routinization stage. Based on this information about the process of dissemination of innovation, the question arises of whether or not the ADP staff would in fact want to fully integrate the project within the juvenile court system in its present state.

We describe these issues in the context of this special issue in order to raise these issues within the prevention literature. As Mayer and Davidson (2000) described the barriers facing innovative programs in general, "resistance to change is common and entrenched" (Mayer and Davidson, 2000, p. 433). To date, most of our efforts in the field have been focused on demonstrating the efficacy of our alternative approaches. The experiences described here would indicate that demonstrating program efficacy makes up less than half of the challenges and responsibilities we face. Further, it indicates that our current conceptualization of the prominent dissemination implementation paradigm present clear cut dilemmas for effective preventive alternatives.

IMPLICATIONS FOR FUTURE RESEARCH

The challenge highlighted here is that future prevention research must move beyond only consideration of model development and include scientific inquiry into understanding how effective preventive models can survive. There is little doubt that future work will need to include additional levels of analysis beyond individual outcomes in order to understand these processes. Individual outcomes and cost, while important, may not be a strong enough armamentarium for the task at hand. While this type of research would expand our knowledge of community impact, alternative prevention programs would still face the challenges of being an "alternative" to a pre-established system, as outlined by the discussion of dissemination of innovation. It is the hope that by providing evidence of individual outcomes across multiple domains and beginning to understand the complexities of long term survival, effective prevention programs may continue to sustain themselves.

REFERENCES

Angelique, H. L., Reischl, T. M., & Davidson, W. S. II. (2002). Promoting political empowerment. *American Journal of Community Psychology, 30*(6), 815-833.

Becker, H. S. (1963) *Outsiders: Studies in the sociology of deviance.* New York: Free Press.

Blakely C., Mayer, J., Gottahalk, R., Schmitt, N., Davidson, W. Roitmen, D., & Emshoff, J. (1987). The fidelity-adaptation debate: Implications for the implementation of public sector social programs. *American Journal of Community Psychology, 15,* 253-268.

Davidson, W. S., & Basta, J. (1989). Diversion from the juvenile justice system: Research evidence and discussion of issues. In B. Lahey & A. Kazdin (Eds.), *Advances in clinical psychology, 12,* 85-112. New York: Plenum Publishing Corporation.

Davidson, W. S. II., Jefferson, S. D., Legaspi, A., Lujan, J., & Wolf, A. M. (2000). Alternative interventions for juvenile offenders: History of the Adolescent Diversion Project. In C. R. Hollin (Ed.), *Handbook of offender assessment and treatment* (pp. 221-236). New York: John Wiley & Sons Ltd.

Davidson, W. S. II, & Johnson, C. (1986). Diversion in Michigan. Lansing, MI: Department of Social Services, Office of Children and Youth Services.

Davidson, W. S. II, & Rapp, C. (1976). Child advocacy in the justice system. *Social Work, 21*(3), 225-232.

Davidson, W. S. II, & Redner, R. (1988). The prevention of juvenile delinquency: Diversion from the juvenile justice system. In R. Price, E. Cowen, R. Lorion, & J. Ramos-McKay (Eds.), *Fourteen ounces of prevention* (pp. 123-137). Washington, DC: American Psychological Association.

Davidson, W. S., Redner, R., Blakely, C. H., Mitchell, C. M., & Emshoff, J. G. (1987). Diversion of juvenile offenders: An experimental comparison. *Journal of Consulting and Clinical Psychology, 55,* 68-75.

Davidson, W. S. II, Redner, R., Amdur, R. L., & Mitchell, C. M. (1990). *Alternative treatments for troubled youth: The case of diversion from the justice system.* New York: Plenum Press.

Davidson, W. S., & Seidman, E. (1974). Studies of behavior modification and juvenile delinquency: A review, methodological critique, and social perspective. *Psychological Bulletin, 81,* 998-1011

Davidson, W. S. II, Seidman, E., Rappaport, J., Berck, P. L., Rapp, N. A., Rhodes, W., & Herring, J. (1977). Diversion program for juvenile offenders. *Social Work Research and Abstracts, 13*(2), 40-49.

Fairweather, G. W., & Davidson, W. S. II. (1986). *An introduction to community experimentation: Theory methods and practice.* New York, NY: McGraw-Hill.

Fairweather, G. W., & Tornatzky, L. G. (1977). *Experimental methods for social policy.* New York: Pergamon.

Gensheimer, L. K. (1987). *Training paraprofessionals: Comparison of two instructional methods used in a paraprofessional diversion program for juvenile delinquents.* Unpublished doctoral dissertation, Michigan State University, East Lansing.

Gensheimer, L. K., Mayer, J. P., Gottschalk, R., & Davidson, W. S. II. (1986). Diverting youth from the juvenile justice system: A meta-analysis of intervention efficacy. In S. J. Apter & A. P. Goldstein (Eds.), *Youth violence: Programs & prospects* (pp. 39-57). New York: Pergamon Press.

Gold, M. (1974). *A time for skepticism.* Belmont, CA: Brooks/Cole.

Ingham County. (2002). Juvenile millage approved by voters. Retrieved September 4, 2003 from *http://www.ingham.org.*

Klein, M. (1979). Deinstitutionalization and diversion of juvenile offenders: A litany of impediments. In N. Morris & M. Tonry (Eds.), *Crime and justice: An annual review of research.* Chicago: University of Chicago Press.

Krisberg, B & Austin, J. (1978) *The children of Ishmael.* Palo Alto, CA: Mayfield Press.

Lipsey, M. W. (1992). Juvenile delinquency treatment: A meta-analytic inquiry into the variability of effects. In T. D. Cook, H. Cooper, D. S. Cordray, H. Hartmann, L. V. Hedges, & R. J. Light et al. (Eds.), *Meta analysis for explanation: A casebook* (pp. 83-127). New York: Russell Sage Foundation.

Mayer, J. P., & Davidson, W. S. II. (2000). Dissemination of innovation as social change. In J. Rappaport and E. Seidman (Eds.), *Handbook of community psychology* (pp. 421-438). New York, NY: Kluwer Academic/Plenum Publishers.

Mitchell, C. M. (1990). *Nonprofessionals working with delinquent youth: An experimental comparison of university, community college and community nonprofessionals.* Unpublished doctoral dissertation, Michigan State University, East Lansing.

Patterson, G. R. (1971). *Raising children.* Champaign, IL: Research Press.

President's Commission on Law Enforcement and the Administration of Justice. (1967). *Juvenile delinquency and youth crime.* Washington, DC: U.S. Government Printing Office.

Rappaport, J., Chinsky, J. & Cowen, E. L. (1971). *Innovations in helping chronic mental patients: College students in a mental institution.* New York: Holt.

Shelden, R. G. (1999). Detention diversion advocacy: An evaluation. *Juvenile Justice Bulletin, September,* 1-15.

Smith, E. P., Wolf, A. M., Cantillon, D. M., Thomas, O., & Davidson, W. S. II. Smith, E. P., (2004). The Adolescent Diversion Project: 25 years of research on an ecological model of intervention. *Journal of Prevention & Intervention in the Community, 27*(2), 29-47.

Tharp, R. L., & Wetzel, R. (1969) *Behavior modification in the natural environment.* New York: Academic

Yin, R. K. (1977). Production efficiency versus bureaucratic self-interest: Two innovative processes? *Policy Sciences, 8,* 381-389.

APPENDIX

Bibliography: Past Studies Showing the Efficacy of the Adolescent Diversion Project

Basta, J. M., & Davidson, W. S. (1988). Treatment of juvenile offenders: Study outcomes since 1980. *Behavioral Sciences & the Law, 6*, 355-384.

Bauer, M., Bordeaux, G., Cole, J., Davidson, W. S., Martinez, A., Mitchell, C. M., & Singleton, D. (1980). A diversion program for juvenile offenders: The experience of Ingham County, Michigan. *Journal of Juvenile and Family Courts, 31*, 53-62.

Blakely, C. H., & Davidson, W. S. (1982). Behavioral approaches to delinquency: A review. In P. Karoly (Ed.), *Adolescent behavior disorders: Current perspectives.* New York: Pergamon.

Blakely, C. H., Kushler, M. G., Parisian, J. A., & Davidson, W. S. (1980). Self-reported estimates of delinquency: Comparative reliability and validity of alternative weighting schemes. *Criminal Justice and Behavior, 7*(4), 369-386.

Davidson, W. S. (1975). The Champaign-Urbana diversion project. *Policeman*, 6-25.

Davidson, W. S., & Basta, J. (1989). Diversion from the juvenile justice system: Research evidence and discussion of issues. In B. Lahey & A. Kazdin (Eds.), *Advances in clinical psychology, 12*, 85-112. New York: Plenum Publishing Corporation.

Davidson, W. S., Gensheimer, L. K., Mayer, J., & Gottschalk, R. (1988). Current status of rehabilitation programs for juvenile offenders. In C. Hampton (Ed.), *Antisocial behavior and substance abuse.* Washington, DC: U.S. Government Printing.

Davidson, W. S., Gottschalk, R., Gensheimer, L., & Mayer, J. (1985). Intervention with juvenile delinquents: A meta-analysis of treatment efficiency. In NIJ/NIMH, *Current status of research in juvenile justice.* Washington, DC: U.S. Government Printing Office.

Davidson, W.S. II, Jefferson, S.D., Legaspi, A., Lujan, J., and Wolf A.M. (2000) Alternative Interventions for Juvenile Offenders: History of the Adolescent Diversion Project. In C.R. Hollin (Ed.) *Handbook of offender assessment and treatment*, New York: Wiley.

Davidson, W. S., & Rapp, C. A. (1976). A multiple strategy model of child advocacy: Implications for the juvenile justice system. *Social Work, 21*, 225-232.

Davidson, W. S., & Redner, R. (1988). The prevention of juvenile delinquency: Diversion from the juvenile justice system. In R. Price, E. Cowen, R. Lorion, & J. Ramos-McKay (Eds.), *14 ounces of prevention.* Washington, DC: APA.

Davidson, W. S., Redner, R., Blakely, C. H., Mitchell, C. M., & Emshoff, J. G. (1987). Diversion of juvenile offenders: An experimental comparison. *Journal of Consulting and Clinical Psychology, 55*, 68-75.

Davidson, W. S., Redner, R., Mitchell, C. M., & Amdur, R. (1990). *Alternative treatments for troubled youth.* New York: Plenum.

Davidson, W. S., & Saul, J. (1982). Child advocacy in the juvenile court: A clash of paradigms. In G. Melton (Ed.), *Legal reforms affecting child and youth services.* New York: The Haworth Press, Inc.

Davidson, W. S., & Seidman, E. (with Abt Associates Staff) (1975). *Exemplary project screening and validation reports: Community-based adolescent diversion project.* Cambridge, MA: Abt Associates.

And reprinted in: R. Ku, K. Bleu, with the assistance of J. Rappaport, E. Seidman, & W. S. Davidson (1977). *Out of the ivory tower: A university's approach to delinquency prevention.* Washington, DC: U.S. Department

Davidson, W. S., Seidman, E., Rappaport, J., Berck, P., Rapp, N., Rhodes, W., & Herring, J. (1977). Diversion programs for juvenile offenders. *Social Work Research and Abstracts, 13*, 41-49.

This work summarized in: Seidman, E., Rappaport, J., & Davidson, W. S. (1976). Diversion programs for juvenile offenders. *Consulting Psychologist Newsletter, 21*, 13-16.

Davidson, W. S., Snellman, L., & Koch, J. R. (1981). Current status of diversion research: Implications for policy and programming. In R. Roesch & R. Corrado (Eds.), *Evaluation and criminal justice policy.* Beverly Hills: Sage.

Eby, K. K., Mackin, J. R., Scofield, M. G., Legler, R. E., & Davidson, W. S. II (1995). The Adolescent Diversion Project. In R. R. Ross (Ed.), *Going Straight: Effective Delinquency Prevention and Offender Rehabilitation.* Ottawa, Canada: Air Training and Publication.

Gensheimer, L. K., Davidson, W. S., Mayer, J., & Gottschalk, R. (1986). Analysis of diversion programs for juvenile delinquents. In A. Goldstein & S. Apter (Eds.), *Youth Violence.* New York: Pergamon.

Gottschalk, R., Davidson, W. S., Gensheimer, L. K., & Mayer, J. (1988). Community based interventions with juvenile delinquents. In H. C. Quay (Ed.), *Handbook of juvenile delinquency.* New York: Wiley.

Kantrowitz, R., Mitchell, C. M., & Davidson, W. S. (1982). Varying formats of teaching undergraduate field courses: An experimental examination. *Teaching of Psychology, 9*, 186-189.

Legler, R. E., Schillo, B. A., Speth, T., & Davidson, W. S. (1996). Prevention and diversion programs. In C. R. Hollin & K. Howells (Eds.), *Clinical approaches to working with young offenders* (pp. 109-125). New York: Wiley.

Mackin, J. R., Eby, K. K., Scofield, M.G., & Davidson, W. S. II (1999). Integrating the ivory tower and the community: The adolescent diversion project. In J. P. McKinney, L. B. Schiamberg, & L. Shelton (Eds.), *Teaching the course on adolescent development.*

Mayer, J., Gensheimer, L. K., Gottschalk, R., & Davidson, W. S. (1986). Current status of behavioral interventions with juvenile offenders. In A. Goldstein & S. Apter (Eds.), *Youth Violence.* New York: Pergamon.

McVeigh, J., Davidson, W. S., & Redner, R. (1984). The long term impact of nonprofessional service experience on college students. *American Journal of Community Psychology, 12*, 725-729.

Mitchell, C. M., Davidson, W. S., Chodakowski, J. A., & McVeigh, J. (1985). Intervention orientation: Quantification of "person blame" versus "situation blame" intervention philosophies. *American Journal of Community Psychology, 13*, 543-552.

Mitchell, C. M., Davidson, W. S., Redner, R., Blakely, C., & Emshoff, J. (1985). Nonprofessional counselors: Revisiting selection and impact issues. *American Journal of Community Psychology, 13*, 203-220.

Mitchell, C. M., Kantrowitz, R., & Davidson, W. S. (1980). Differential attitude change in nonprofessional experience: An experimental comparison. *Journal of Counseling Psychology*, *27*(6), 625-629.

Redner, R., Snellman, L., & Davidson, W. S. (1983). Review of behavior methods in the treatment of delinquents. In R. J. Morris & T. R. Kratochwill (Eds.), *Practice of therapy with children: A textbook of methods*. New York: Pergamon.

Schillo, B. A. & Davidson, W. S. II (1994). The need for alternatives to secure detention for juvenile offenders. *Journal for Juvenile Justice and Detention Services*, *9*, 7-16.

Scofield, M. E., & Davidson, W. S. (1999). Community approaches to delinquency control. In A. Goldstein (Ed.). *Effective correctional practice*, New York: American Correctional Association

Smith, E., Wolf, A. M., Cantillon, D. M., Thomas, O., & Davidson, W. S. (2004) The Adolescent Diversion Project: 25 years of research on an ecological model of intervention. *Journal of Prevention & Intervention in the Community*, 29-47.

Assessment of Home-Based Behavior Modification Programs for Autistic Children: Reliability and Validity of the Behavioral Summarized Evaluation

Brent J. Oneal
Roger N. Reeb
John R. Korte
Eliot J. Butter

University of Dayton

SUMMARY. Since the publication of Lovaas' (1987) impressive findings, there has been a proliferation of home-based behavior modification programs for autistic children. Parents and other paraprofessionals often play key roles in the implementation and monitoring of these programs. The Behavioral Summarized Evaluation (BSE) was developed for professionals and paraprofessionals to use in assessing the severity of autistic symptoms over the course of treatment. This paper examined the psychometric properties of the BSE (inter-item consistency, factorial composition, convergent validity, and sensitivity to parents' perceptions

---

Address correspondence to: Roger N. Reeb, Department of Psychology, University of Dayton, Dayton, OH 45469-1430 (E-mail: roger.reeb@notes.udayton.edu).

The authors wish to thank David W. Biers, Department of Psychology, University of Dayton, for his helpful suggestions regarding data analysis.

This research is based on a masters thesis completed by the first author under the second author's supervision.

[Haworth co-indexing entry note]: "Assessment of Home-Based Behavior Modification Programs for Autistic Children: Reliability and Validity of the Behavioral Summarized Evaluation." Oneal et al. Co-published simultaneously in *Journal of Prevention & Intervention in the Community* (The Haworth Press, Inc.) Vol. 32, No. 1/2, 2006, pp. 25-39 and: *Community Action Research: Benefits to Community Members and Service Providers* (ed: Roger N. Reeb) The Haworth Press, Inc., 2006, pp. 25-39. Single or multiple copies of this article are available for a fee from The Haworth Document Delivery Service [1-800-HAWORTH, 9:00 a.m. - 5:00 p.m. (EST). E-mail address: docdelivery@haworthpress.com].

of symptom change over time) when used by parents of autistic youngsters undergoing home-based intervention. Recommendations for future
research are presented. *[Article copies available for a fee from The Haworth
Document Delivery Service: 1-800-HAWORTH. E-mail address: <docdelivery@
haworthpress.com> Website: <http://www.HaworthPress.com> © 2006 by The
Haworth Press, Inc. All rights reserved.]*

KEYWORDS. Autism, home-based treatment, behavior therapy, behavior modification, assessment, Behavioral Summarized Evaluation

As defined by the American Psychiatric Association (2000), the essential features of autism, which has an onset prior to the age of 3 years,
include: qualitative impairment in social interaction (e.g., lack of social
or emotional reciprocity), qualitative impairment in communication
(e.g., delay or lack of speech or echolalia), and markedly restricted, re-
petitive, and stereotyped patterns of behavior, motor mannerisms
(e.g., hand flapping), interests, and activities. The use of behavior
modification for autism has become increasingly common (Johnson & Hastings, 2002), and this treatment approach is based on the
rationale that " . . . autism is a syndrome of behavioral deficits and ex-
cesses that have a neurological basis, but are nonetheless amenable to
change in response to specific, carefully programmed, constructive interactions with the environment" (Green, 1996, p. 30). This study further examined the reliability and validity of the Behavioral Summarized
Evaluation (BSE; Barthelemy et al., 1990), which was developed for
professionals and paraprofessionals to use in assessing the severity of
autistic symptoms over the course of treatment.

BACKGROUND

Discussion regarding the implementation and assessment of behavior modification programs for autistic children tends to center around
the research published by Ivar Lovaas at the University of California,
Los Angeles (UCLA). Therefore, a brief review of the UCLA Young
Autism Project is necessary in order to provide a context for the findings presented in this article.

In a classic study by Lovaas (1987), autistic children were assigned
to one of two groups: (a) an intensive-treatment group ($n = 19$), which
received more than 40 hours of one-to-one treatment per week; or (b) a
minimal-treatment control group ($n = 19$), which received 10 hours or

less of one-to-one treatment per week. In this study, the children were below the age of 4 years, and the autism diagnosis was made by a clinician who was independent from the study. Random assignment was not employed due to "parent protest and ethical considerations" (Lovaas, 1987, p. 4), and group assignment was dependent on "the number of staff members available to render treatment." Nevertheless, the researchers did show that the two groups were similar on numerous pre-treatment measures. Both groups received treatment for 2 or more years. The conceptual basis for the behavior modification was reinforcement (operant) theory. As Lovaas (1987, p. 3) noted, the general plan is for autistic children to receive the behavioral treatment "during most of their waking hours for many years," with treatment involving " . . . all significant persons in all significant environments." To guard against the possibility that autistic children referred to Lovaas' program represented a subgroup with particularly "favorable" or "unfavorable" outcomes, a second control group ($n = 21$) of autistic children from a different study was also employed.

Follow-up results indicated that 9 of the children (47%) in the intensive treatment group obtained an IQ score in the average or above average range and exhibited successful performance in a regular first grade class in public school. Eight children (42%) in the intensive treatment group obtained IQ scores in the mildly mentally retarded range and attended special classes for language delay, while only 2 children (10%) had IQ scores in the profoundly mentally retarded range and attended special classes for autistic/mentally retarded children. The two minimal treatment control groups did not differ significantly at pre-treatment or at follow-up. In contrast to the follow-up results for the intensive treatment group, only one participant (2%) in the minimal treatment control groups obtained an IQ score in the average range and was placed in regular first-grade class in public school. Furthermore, 18 of the children in the control groups (45%) had IQ scores in mildly mentally retarded range and were placed in classes for language delay, and 21 of the children (53%) had IQ scores in the severely mentally retarded range and were placed in autistic/mentally retarded classes. A long-term follow-up study (McEachin, Smith, & Lovaas, 1993), in which the ages of children ranged from 9 to 19 years, found that treatment gains were generally maintained. For instance, among the 9 children who achieved normal functioning by age 7 and ended treatment at that point, 8 were " . . . able to hold their own in the regular classroom, did not show signs of emotional disturbance, and demonstrated adequate . . . adaptive and social skills within the normal range" (McEachin et al., 1993, p. 368).

The findings published by Lovaas' research group are controversial, as illustrated by the debate between Gresham and MacMillan (1997) and Smith and Lovaas (1997). Lovaas and colleagues have expressed caution about unwarranted generalizations regarding their initial findings: "Even though the results to date on the effectiveness of intensive early intervention are very encouraging, these results and procedures must be replicated by independent researchers before intensive early intervention can be given widespread endorsement" (Lovaas & Buch, 1997, p. 82). Systematic replications by Lovaas and colleagues (and independent researchers) have been underway on a national and international level (see www.lovaas.com/index.html; Sallows & Graupner, 1999), and the preliminary results have been impressive.

One notable outcome of Lovaas' research is the proliferation of home-based behavior modification programs for autistic children. In Lovaas' (1987, p. 5) original paper, it was emphasized that " . . . parents worked as part of the treatment team . . . " and that parents were "extensively trained in the treatment procedures so that treatment could take place for almost all of the subjects' waking hours, 365 days a year." After discussing the literature, Schreibman (2000, p. 375) concluded: "More extensive generalization and better maintenance of treatment effects are achieved when parents are trained to be major treatment providers."

In home-based programs, parents, students, and other paraprofessionals often receive training in Lovaas' methods (see teaching manuals by: Lovaas, 2003; Lovaas et al., 1980) and play major roles in implementing the treatment. Typically, an expert consultant supervises and oversees the treatment program. A literature review suggests that there is significant variability among studies regarding the intensity of home-based treatment, the level of supervision of parents, students, and paraprofessionals, the number of therapists involved, and the extent to which other community services are available. As an illustration, the reader is encouraged to examine the treatment differences between the study reported by Smith, Groen, and Wynn (2000) and the study by Sheinkopf and Siegel (1998). It appears that the inconsistency in these treatment variables may be even greater among the home-based treatment programs that are parent-managed (see a review by Mudford, Martin, Eikeseth, & Bibby, 2001). Further, as noted by Johnson and Hastings (2002, p. 123), " . . . international interest in intensive home-based early behavioral intervention for children with autism is increasing," but " . . . there is little or no published research on the experiences of [these] families. . . . " One concern involves the ways in which parents monitor the child's progress in response to treatment. While inconsistency across published studies regarding strategies for outcome assessment is a general concern in research on behavioral treatment for autistic children (Schreibman, 2000), a lack of consistent and systematic use of well-validated assessment procedures may represent a particular problem in parent-managed programs (see Mudford et al., 2002).

THE PRESENT STUDY

Given the high level of parent involvement in home-based behavior modification programs for autistic children, a reliable and valid psychometric instrument that can be used by parents and other paraprofessionals in monitoring progress is needed. Thus, the purpose of the present study was to further examine the reliability and validity of the Behavioral Summarized Evaluation (BSE; Barthelemy et al., 1990). The BSE, which was initially developed by Lelord et al. (1981) and later examined and modified by Barthelemy and colleagues (1990, 1992, 1997), evaluates the severity of behavioral problems in autistic children. More specifically, Barthelemy and colleagues have noted that the BSE was developed for the following purpose: (a) to "evaluate the severity of behavioral problems in autistic children" (1992, p. 29); and (b) to "measure changes of behavioral parameters over time and treatments . . . " (1990, p. 195). With regard to practical considerations, the instrument was intentionally developed to be (a) " . . . simple, quick to administer" (1992, p. 23) and (b) " . . . easy to handle and accessible to professionals and paraprofessionals . . . " (1990, p. 190).

In the Bartelemy et al. (1990) study, the kappa statistic indicated "excellent" interrater reliability for two items (.75-1.00), "good" reliability for twelve items (.60-.74), and "fair" reliability for five items (.40-.59). Using the intraclass correlation, these researchers reported "excellent" interrater reliability (.96) for the global score. Barthelemy et al. (1997) reported similar evidence of interrater reliability. With regard to content validity, a factor analysis of BSE items conducted by Barthelemy et al. (1990) produced six factors with eigenvalues of at least 1, with two primary factors cumulatively accounting for 43.7% of the total variance. Barthelemy et al. (1997) reported similar factor analytic findings. Regarding criterion-related validity, Barthelemy et al. (1990, 1997) found that Factor 1 of the BSE significantly correlated with Expert Severity Scores provided by experienced clinicians. Given the importance of

Factor 1, the researchers have labeled it "Autism" (Barthelemy et al., 1990, p. 192) or "Interaction Disorder" (Barthelemy et al., 1997, p. 145). Concerning convergent validity, Barthelemy et al. (1992) demonstrated that the BSE effectively discriminated between children diagnosed with Autistic Disorder versus Mental Retardation, and Barthelemy et al. (1997) found that the BSE discriminated among children diagnosed with Autistic Disorder from those diagnosed with either Mental Retardation or Pervasive Developmental Disorder Not Otherwise Specified. Finally, Barthelemy et al. (1997) reported preliminary data suggesting that BSE ratings change in the hypothesized direction in response to intervention. That is, for a group of eight autistic youngsters receiving behavior therapy, BSE rating scores obtained monthly improved systematically over a 9-month period.

As a psychometric instrument to be used by parents as well as other paraprofessionals to assist in monitoring autistic symptoms over the course of treatment, the BSE may have a number of practical advantages over other instruments. First, the BSE was specifically designed for use by paraprofessionals or professionals. For instance, each BSE item focuses on a particular autistic symptom and, for each item, clear examples are provided to illustrate the symptom. Second, the BSE is readily available. For instance, the first author of this article was able to obtain permission to use the BSE, free of charge, by faxing a letter to the publishing company outlining the purpose of the study.

METHOD

Participants and Procedures

Participants were 53 primary caregivers (47 mothers, 6 fathers) of autistic children receiving home-based behavior therapy. Participants were recruited by posting a message on an internet listserve dedicated to parents, therapists, and researchers interested in behavior therapy for autistic children. A general description of the study was provided, and interested caregivers were asked to email an address so that a packet of psychometric instruments could be sent to them via regular mail. Using this procedure, 80 packets were mailed out and 53 were returned. The 53 autistic children (43 males, 10 females) ranged in age from 36 months to 127 months ($M = 68.8$ months, $SD = 17.1$). The length of time in home-based behavior therapy ranged from 7 to 62 months ($M = 22.4$ months, $SD = 13.8$ months).

Description of the Home-Based Behavior Modification

Consistent with other studies in this area (see Johnson & Hastings, 2002; Mudford et al., 2001), there was variability among families with regard to treatment intensity and number of therapists involved. However, there were three common factors among the treatment regimes. First, each parent reported that, in general, the home-based behavior modification was modeled after the Lovaas treatment program (see teaching manuals by: Lovaas, 2003; Lovaas, Ackerman, Alexander, Firestone, Perkins, & Young, 1981). Second, there was evidence of parental involvement in treatment implementation. That is, in response to the question–"To what extent are you involved in providing behavior modification to your child?"–Thirty-one of the parents described themselves as "highly" involved in treatment, and 21 described themselves at least "moderately" involved, with 1 parent only "marginally" involved. Third, each parent reported that a number of therapists were involved during a course of treatment, some of whom were paraprofessionals (e.g., students). Further details regarding the specific treatment program for each child are not available.

Assessment Materials

The packet of psychometric instruments mailed to parents included a basic demographic questionnaire, the BSE, and the Childhood Autism Rating Scale (CARS; Schopler, Reichler, & Renner, 1988). The BSE is a 20-item instrument that examines the scope and severity of behavior problems in autistic children. Each BSE item is scored as 0 (*never*), 1 (*sometimes*), 2 (*often*), 3 (*very often*), or 4 (*always*). A *global score* can be obtained by summing the 20 item scores. The CARS, a well-validated measure of autistic behaviors and characteristics, consists of 15 Likert-like items, each of which assesses the behavioral functioning in an area related to autism. For each item, ratings range from 1 to 4 in .5 increments, with accompanying anchors as follows: 1 (*normal*), 2 (*mildly abnormal*), 3 (*moderately abnormal*), and 4 (*severely abnormal*). As reviewed by Schopler et al. (1980, 1988), there is excellent evidence of reliability and validity for the CARS. Although the CARS was designed to be used by trained professionals, Bebko, Konstantareas, and Springer (1987) found that parents may be able to use the CARS in a meaningful way if it is modified by excluding the "general impressions" category.

RESULTS AND DISCUSSION

Inter-Item Consistency

The caregivers' retrospective ratings on the BSE (based on memory of autistic symptoms prior to home-based behavior therapy) indicated a high level of inter-item consistency (Cronbach's alpha coefficient = .83). Individual item analysis indicated that none of the items detracted from the level of inter-item consistency (alpha coefficient). The caregivers' current ratings on the BSE (based on perceptions of autistic symptoms at present) also revealed a high level of inter-item consistency (Cronbach's alpha coefficient = .90), again with none of the items detracting from the level of inter-item consistency. Thus, when parents use the BSE, it continues to have excellent inter-item consistency.

Construct Validity: Factorial Composition

As expected, there are similarities between the factor analysis results of the present study (with parents as evaluators) and those of the original Barthelemy et al. (1990) study (using professionals as raters). First, consistent with the Barthelemy et al. (1990) study, the factor analysis produced six factors with eigenvalues greater than 1, and two main factors cumulatively accounting for over 42.1% of the variance. Table 1 reports the eigenvalues and the percentage of variance accounted for by each of the six factors in the present study and in the original research by Barthelemy et al. (1990). Second, there is a great deal of similarity between the two studies regarding the actual item loadings for Factor 1, which has been labeled "Autism" (Barthelemy et al., 1990, p. 192) or "Interaction Disorder" (Barthelemy et al., 1997, p. 145). Table 2 provides BSE item loadings on Factor 1 for the present study, as well as the original factor analytic study by Barthelemy et al. (1990). As Table 2 illustrates, five items (1, 2, 3, 6, and 19) out of the seven items that loaded (> .60) on Factor 1 in the original Barthelemy et al. (1990) study also loaded on Factor 1 in the present study. As noted earlier, Factor 1 appears to be by far the most important factor, since it is the only factor to correlate with independent (blind) criteria, including the Expert Severity Scores provided by experienced clinicians (Barthelemy et al., 1990, 1997) and the Rimland (1971) E2 Diagnostic Checklist (Barthelemy et al., 1997). With regard to items 4 and 20, the only two items found to load on Factor 2 by Barthelemy et al. (1990) but not by the present study, parents and professionals may differ in their ability to detect or

TABLE 1. Eigenvalues and Percentage of the Variance Accounted for the Six BSE Factors in the Present Study and the Barthelemy et al. (1990) Study

Factor	Eigenvalue		% of Variance	
	Present Study	Barthelemy et al. 1990	Present Study	Barthelemy et al. 1990
1	5.77	6.08	28.9	30.4
2	2.64	2.67	13.2	13.3
3	1.51	1.65	7.6	8.2
4	1.45	1.38	7.3	6.9
5	1.23	1.16	6.2	5.8
6	1.03	1.05	5.1	5.2

judge the severity of these symptoms, and further research would be needed to understand this pattern. In sum, the similarity of the factor analytic findings of Barthelemy et al. (1990) and those of the present study suggest that parents and professionals are judging BSE items in similar ways. This provides some justification for the use of the BSE by parents involved in the treatment team, though further research is needed to determine the utility of this assessment component.

In general, based on the factor analysis results of this study, the study by Barthelemy et al. (1990), and the study by Barthelemy et al. (1997), there appears to be considerable inconsistency regarding which BSE items load on Factor 2. Barthelemy et al. (1997) found three items to load on Factor 2, but none of these items loaded on Factor 2 in the Barthelemy et al. (1990) study nor in the present study. Barthelemy et al. (1990) had found two other items to load on Factor 2, but neither of these items loaded on Factor 2 in the Barthelemy et al. (1997) study, and only one of them (item 13) loaded on Factor 2 in the present study. The present study also found three other items (items 4, 11, 20) that loaded on Factor 2, but none of these items loaded on Factor 2 in the studies by Barthelemy et al. (1990, 1997). Further, Barthelemy et al. (1997) have questioned the utility of Factor 2 because it "is not correlated with" independent criteria (p. 150). Barthelemy et al. (1997, p. 150) note that Factor 2 " . . . comprises symptoms not directly involved with autistic syndrome but which may be associated with it." Thus, further research is needed to determine the validity and practical utility of Factor 2.

TABLE 2. BSE Item Loadings on Factor 1 for the Present Study and the Original Factor Analytic Study by Barthelemy et al. (1990)

BSE Item	Present Study	Barthelemy et al. 1990
1. Is eager for aloneness	**.79**	**.84**
2. Ignores people	**.70**	**.88**
3. Poor social interaction	**.80**	**.61**
4. Abnormal eye contact	.36	**.77**
5. Does not make an effort to communicate using voice and/or words	.23	.41
6. Lack of appropriate facial expression and gestures	**.67**	**.70**
7. Stereotyped vocal and voice utterances, echolalia	.01	.11
8. Lack of initiative, poor activity	.23	.45
9. Inappropriate relating to inanimate objects or to a doll	.32	.25
10. Resistance to change and to frustration	.05	.06
11. Stereotyped sensorimotor activity	.12	.56
12. Agitation, restlessness	.16	.09
13. Bizarre posture and gait	.30	.25
14. Auto-aggressiveness	−.10	.00
15. Heteroaggressiveness	−.14	**−.19**
16. Soft anxiety signs	.01	.14
17. Mood difficulties	.27	.04
18. Disturbance of feeding behavior	.15	.09
19. Unstable attention, easily distracted	**.64**	**.64**
20. Bizarre responses to auditory stimuli	.15	**.73**

Note. When an item loading is in *bold*, this indicates that the item loaded heavily on Factor 1.

Construct Validity: Sensitivity to Perceptions of Behavioral Change Over Time

One important issue in construct validity involves the extent to which there is evidence that scores on an instrument change in the hypothesized direction over the course of an intervention (Anastasi & Urbina, 1997; Cronbach & Meehl, 1955). Given that home-based behavior therapy has been shown to benefit autistic children, caregivers' current BSE ratings were expected to be significantly lower than caregivers' retrospective BSE ratings. As noted by Barthelemy et al. (1990), preliminary evidence suggests that the BSE is sensitive to behavioral changes during therapeutic trials, but it "is also necessary to confirm statistically that the BSE is sensitive enough to show clinically significant changes in behavior over time" (p. 196). As expected, the difference between caregivers' retrospective BSE ratings ($M = 46.87$, $SD = 9.68$) and current BSE ratings ($M = 17.97$, $SD = 9.68$) was statistically significant, $t(52) = -18.81$, $p = .001$. When the psychometric properties of an instrument are examined, it is important to determine if the expected pattern is observed for each item (Anastasi & Urbina, 1997). As illustrated in Table 3, the difference between retrospective and current BSE ratings was significant for every BSE item. These results suggest that the BSE is sensitive to behavioral changes that occur over the course of home-based behavior modification.

Although parents' BSE ratings revealed a perceived decrease in autistic symptoms over the course of treatment, some degree of consistency in ranking across retrospective and current ratings was expected and observed. That is, results indicated a significant correlation between BSE retrospective and current ratings ($r = .42$, $p = .002$), with the correlation coefficient ranging from .37 ($p < .004$) to .69 ($p < .001$) across the 20 BSE items.

Construct Validity: Convergent Validation

To determine convergent validity (Campbell & Fiske, 1959), the relationship between the BSE and the CARS (Schopler et al., 1988), another well-validated measure of autism, was examined. The correlation coefficient between the BSE and the CARS total scores was high in magnitude and significant across caregivers' retrospective ratings ($r = .80$, $p = .001$) and caregivers' current ratings ($r = .84$, $p = .001$). Further, the correlation coefficient between the difference scores for the BSE and CARS (i.e., difference between caregivers' retrospective and current ratings) was high in magnitude and significant ($r = .77$, $p = .001$), suggesting that the level of caregivers' per-

TABLE 3. Means and Standard Deviations for BSE Retrospective and Current Ratings (N = 53)

BSE Item	Retrospective		Current			
	M	SD	M	SD	t-value	p-value
1. Is eager for aloneness	3.19	.74	1.23	.67	−18.23	.001
2. Ignores people	2.91	.84	.87	.71	−17.37	.001
3. Poor social interaction	3.30	.72	1.15	.86	−17.68	.001
4. Abnormal eye contact	2.91	.95	1.04	.73	−14.77	.001
5. Does not make an effort to communicate using voice and/or words	2.91	1.04	.64	.86	−13.79	.001
6. Lack of appropriate facial expression and gestures	2.45	1.12	.51	.64	−14.31	.001
7. Stereotyped vocal and voice utterances, echolalia	2.57	1.34	1.13	.96	−6.09	.001
8. Lack of initiative, poor activity	3.19	1.04	1.36	1.13	−11.70	.001
9. Inappropriate relating to inanimate objects or to a doll	2.72	1.23	.87	.92	−13.36	.001
10. Resistance to change and to frustration	2.57	1.31	1.06	.80	−9.02	.001
11. Stereotyped sensorimotor activity	2.09	1.17	.98	.84	−8.32	.001
12. Agitation, restlessness	2.02	1.39	1.09	.93	−5.18	.001
13. Bizarre posture and gait	1.23	1.10	.58	.63	−5.31	.001
14. Auto-aggressiveness	.98	1.17	.36	.59	−4.28	.001
15. Heteroaggressiveness	1.08	1.25	.60	.69	−2.89	.001
16. Soft anxiety signs	1.34	1.24	.72	.82	−5.02	.001
17. Mood difficulties	1.81	1.09	.81	.71	−7.14	.001
18. Disturbance of feeding behavior	1.92	1.44	.96	1.13	−6.22	.001
19. Unstable attention, easily distracted	2.92	1.02	1.02	.69	−14.36	.001
20. Bizarre responses to auditory stimuli	2.72	1.15	.89	.75	−12.46	.001

Note. df for all analyses was 52.

ceived improvement in autistic symptoms over the course of treatment as indicated by BSE ratings corresponded to the level of perceived improvement based on CARS ratings. This close correspondence between BSE and CARS scores suggests convergent validity for the BSE as a measure of parents' perceptions of both symptom severity and symptom change.

CONCLUSION

This study suggests that the BSE has acceptable psychometric properties when used by parents to monitor the change in symptoms of autistic children over the course of home-based behavioral treatment. The inter-item consistency of BSE items as completed by parents was found to be excellent. In general, the factor analysis results based on parent BSE ratings in the present study were similar to the factor analysis results of previous studies in which professionals completed BSE ratings (Barthelemy et al., 1990, 1997). Convergent validity was also demonstrated in that BSE ratings correlated highly with ratings on a well-validated psychometric instrument for assessing autistic symptoms (CARS). Further, parents' perceptions of symptom improvements in autistic children over the course of treatment based on BSE ratings (i.e., the difference between retrospective and current BSE ratings) correlated highly with parents' perceptions of symptom improvements based on CARS ratings.

The primary limitations of this study involved the retrospective nature of the research and the lack of an independent expert-based criterion, such as the Expert Severity Scores used by Barthelemy and colleagues (1990, 1997). Therefore, the major research recommendation is a prospective study that systematically examines the correspondence between changes in parents' BSE ratings and changes in experts' ratings over the course of treatment. After implementation of the present study, Barthelemy et al. (1997) revised the BSE by adding several items, and future research should employ the revised version. Since the generalization and maintenance of behavioral treatment effects are enhanced when trained parents are involved in treatment provision (Schreiber, 2000), and given the proliferation of home-based behavior modification program for autistic children (Johnson & Hastings, 2002), a well-validated psychometric instrument appropriate for parent use is needed as one part of a comprehensive (i.e., multidisciplinary and multifaceted) assessment plan. The BSE would appear to be such an instrument.

REFERENCES

American Psychiatric Association (2000). *Diagnostic and Statistical Manual of Mental Disorders*, Fourth Edition, Text Revision. Washington DC: Author.

Anastasi, A. & Urbina, S. (1997). *Psychological Testing* (7th ed.). New Jersey: Prentice Hall.

Barthelemy, C., Adrien, J. L., Roux, S., Garreau, B., Perrot, A., & Lelord, G. (1992). Sensitivity and specificity of the Behavioral Summarized Evaluation (BSE) for the assessment of autistic behaviors. *Journal of Autism and Developmental Disorders, 22*, 23-31.

Barthelemy, C., Adrien, J. L., Tanguay, P., Garreau, B., Fermanian, J., Roux, S., Sauvage, D., & Lelord, G. (1990). The Behavioral Summarized Evaluation: Validity and reliability of a scale for the assessment of autistic behaviors. *Journal of Autism and Developmental Disorders, 20*(2), 189-203.

Barthelemy, C., Roux, S, Adrien, J. L., Hameury, L., Guerin, P., Garreau, B., Fermanian, J., & Lelord, G. (1997). Validation of the Revised Behavior Summarized Evaluation Scale. *Journal of Autism and Developmental Disorders, 27*(2), 139-153.

Bebko, J. M., Konstantareas, M. M., & Springer, J. (1987). Parent and professional evaluations of family stress associated with characteristics of autism. *Journal of Autism and Developmental Disorders, 17*(4), 565-576.

Campbell, D.T., & Fiske, D.W. (1959). Convergent and discriminant validation by the multitrait-multimethod matrix. *Psychological Bulletin, 56*, 81-105.

Cronbach, L.J., & Meehl, P.E. (1955). Construct validity in psychological tests. *Psychological Bulletin, 52*, 281-302.

Green, G. (1996b). Early behavioral intervention for autism: What does research tell us? In Maurice, C. (Ed.), *Behavioral Intervention for Young Children with Autism: A Manual for Parents and Professionals* (pp. 29-44). Austin, TX: PRO-ED.

Gresham, F. M., & MacMillan, D. L. (1997b). Denial and defensiveness in the place of fact and reason: Rejoinder to Smith and Lovaas. *Behavioral Disorders, 4*, 219-230.

Johnson, E., & Hastings, R. P. (2002). Facilitating factors and barriers to the implementation of intensive home-based behavioural intervention for young children with autism. *Child: Care, Health & Development, 28*(2), 123-129.

LeLord, I., Muh, J. P., Barthelemy, C., Martineau, J., Garreau, B, & Callaway, E. (1981). Effects of pyridoxine and magnesium on autistic symptoms. Initial observations. *Journal of Autism and Developmental Disorders, 11*, 219-230.

Lovaas, O. I. (1987). Behavioral treatment and normal educational and intellectual functioning in young autistic children. *Journal of Consulting and Clinical Psychology, 55*, 3-9.

Lovaas, O. I. (2003). *Teaching individuals with developmental delays: Basic intervention techniques*. Austin, TX: PRO-ED.

Lovaas, O. I., Ackerman, A. B., Alexander, D., Firestone, P., Perkins, J., & Young, D. (1980). *Teaching developmentally disabled children: The ME book*. Austin, TX: PRO-ED.

Lovaas, O. I., & Buch, G. (1997). Intensive behavioral intervention with young children with autism. In N. N. Singh (Ed.), *Prevention and treatment of severe behavior problems: Models and methods in developmental disabilities* (pp. 61-86). Pacific Grove, CA: Brooks/Cole.

Lovaas Institute for Early Intervention (LIFE). (n.d.). *Replication Sites.* Retrieved February 9, 2004, from http://www.lovaas.com/index.html.

McEachin, J. J., Smith, T., & Lovaas, O. I. (1993). Long-term outcome for children with autism who received early intensive behavioral treatment. *American Journal of Mental Retardation, 97,* 359-372.

Mudford, O. C., Martin, N. T., Eikeseth, S., & Bibby, P. (2001). Parent-managed behavioral treatment for preschool children with autism: Some characteristics of UK programs. *Research in Developmental Disabilities, 22,* 173-182.

Sallows, G. O., & Graupner, T. D. (1999, June). *Replicating Lovaas' treatment and findings: Preliminary results.* Paper presented at the PEACH Conference, London, England. Retrieved February 9, 2004, from http://www.londonearlyautism.com/Research/research.html.

Schopler, E., Reichler, R. J., Devellis, R. F., & Daly, K. (1980). Toward objective classification of childhood autism: Children Autism Rating Scale (CARS). *Journal of Autism and Developmental Disorders, 10,* 91-103.

Schopler, E. Reichler, R., & Renner, B. (1988). *The Childhood Autism Rating Scale (CARS).* Los Angeles, CA: Western Psychological.

Schreibman, L. (2000). Intensive behavioral/psychoeducational treatments for autism: Research needs and future directions. *Journal of Autism and Developmental Disorders, 30*(5), 373-378.

Sheinkopf, F. J., & Siegel, B. (1998). Home-based behavioral treatment of young autistic children. *Journal of Autism and Developmental Disorders, 28*(1), 15-23.

Smith, T., Groen, A., & Wynn, J. (2000). A randomized trial of intensive early intervention for children. *American Journal on Mental Retardation, 105*(4), 269-285.

Smith, T., & Lovaas, O. I. (1997). The UCLA young autism project: A reply to Gresham and MacMillan. *Behavioral Disorders, 22,* 202-218.

The Tools to Understand:
Community as Co-Researcher
on Culture-Specific Protective Factors
for Alaska Natives

James Allen
University of Alaska Fairbanks, University of Oslo

Gerald V. Mohatt
University of Alaska Fairbanks

S. Michelle Rasmus
University of Alaska Fairbanks

Kelly L. Hazel
Metropolitan State University

Lisa Thomas
University of Washington-Seattle

Sharon Lindley
The PA Team[1]
University of Alaska Fairbanks

Address correspondence to: James Allen, Department of Psychology, University of Alaska Fairbanks, Fairbanks, AK 99775-6480 (E-mail: Jim.Allen@uaf.edu).

The authors would like to thank all of the participants, field interviewers, research assistants, and their coordinating council for their assistance in completing this research.

Research reported in this paper was funded by National Institute of Alcohol Abuse and Alcoholism (NIH) and the National Center for Minority Health Disparities (NCMHD) 1R01 AA 11446-03.

[Haworth co-indexing entry note]: "The Tools to Understand: Community as Co-Researcher on Culture-Specific Protective Factors for Alaska Natives." Allen et al. Co-published simultaneously in *Journal of Prevention & Intervention in the Community* (The Haworth Press, Inc.) Vol. 32, No. 1/2, 2006, pp. 41-59; and: *Community Action Research: Benefits to Community Members and Service Providers* (ed: Roger N. Reeb) The Haworth Press, Inc., 2006, pp. 41-59. Single or multiple copies of this article are available for a fee from The Haworth Document Delivery Service [1-800-HAWORTH, 9:00 a.m. - 5:00 p.m. (EST). E-mail address: docdelivery@haworthpress.com].

SUMMARY. A collaborative research process engaging Alaska Native communities in the study of protective factors in Alaska Native sobriety and the design of a preventative intervention using its findings is described. Study 1 was discovery oriented qualitative research whose objectives were identification of protective factors and development of a heuristic model. Study 2 involved quantitative survey methods to develop and test a measure of protective factors identified by the qualitative study. Empirical data from these studies is presented, and the role of Alaska Native co-researchers who did not possess specialist research training is described in the design and implementation of the study, interpretation of findings, and design of the intervention model and tools. Benefits that emerged from co-researcher involvement in this process, to the community and to the co-researchers themselves, are described. *[Article copies available for a fee from The Haworth Document Delivery Service: 1-800-HAWORTH. E-mail address: <docdelivery@ haworthpress.com> Website: <http://www.HaworthPress.com> © 2006 by The Haworth Press, Inc. All rights reserved.]*

KEYWORDS. Sobriety, American Indian and Alaska Native, alcohol, protective factors, prevention, qualitative methods, participatory action research (PAR)

My father and my mother gave me the tools to understand myself through the teaching they gave us, through the land that we live, and the stars that we have at night, the sun that we have during the day, and all the survival skills.

Yup'ik elder

This article reports on a collaborative research process that engaged Alaska Native communities in an innovative approach to a severe social problem. The People Awakening Project (PA)[1] used participatory action research (PAR) methods (Chesler, 1991; White, Nary, & Froehlich, 2001) to understand sobriety from an Alaska Native perspective, in order to generate knowledge for development of a culturally grounded, multilevel intervention to prevent alcohol use among Alaska Native children. In keeping with the theme of this special volume, our focus is on benefits of this process to communities and our co-researchers, though we also briefly present results identifying protective factors (Rutter, 2000) in sobriety for Alaska Natives. In this paper we use the term "co-researcher"; paraprofessional is a term that offends many Alaska Natives through its emphasis on Western education as sole means of credentialing, recalling a rhetoric of colonialism. PA co-researchers were Alaska Natives who, despite not possessing four-year university degrees or research training, brought to PA rich knowledge of their culture and the sobriety process. PA co-researchers worked collaboratively with university researchers as a coordinating council co-directing the project, and as research staff, field workers, cultural consultants, and translators.

THE ALASKA NATIVE RURAL CONTEXT

Though often viewed from outside Alaska as a single group, Alaska Natives comprise over 225 federally recognized tribes often combined into five major cultural groups: in the north, the Inupiaq; in the interior of Alaska, the Athabascan; in the southwest, the Yup'ik and Cup'ik; in the south and west along the coast and Aleutians, the Aleut and the Alutiiq; and to the southeast, the Tlingit, Haida, and Tsimshian. Each group engages in unique subsistence economies, cultural practices, and rituals. Linguistically, the indigenous languages can differ as much as English and Chinese, in that they represent entirely distinct language families. Within groups, significant cultural diversity also exists; for example, there are at least 11 recognized regional dialects of Athabascan. PA studied sobriety among all five groups, and the prevention intervention described in this paper is for use with the largest, the Yup'ik.

Though almost half of Alaska Natives reside in urban centers, the majority live in widely dispersed rural villages where they typically comprise the majority ethnic group. These villages rarely have road access, and can be several hours from urban centers by small plane. Most cash economy work is limited to education, health care, and government, with some seasonal employment opportunities in construction, fire fighting, tourism, and natural resources management. The majority of rural residents maintain a subsistence way of life through hunting and gathering that provides the major portion of their diet, as well as being culturally and spiritually significant. Distance and isolation are factors in the maintenance of a distinct cultural identity during a period of recent and rapid social transition. In the Yup'ik, as well as in some of the other cultural groups, several communities have adopted a language immersion education model. In many Yup'ik villages the indigenous language is the first language.

ALASKA NATIVE SOBRIETY AND PA

Alcohol abuse has devastating health and social consequences for many Alaska Natives. Cirrhosis death rates for Alaska Natives were 18.7 per 100,000, in contrast to the U.S. baseline of 9.6, and alcohol is linked to 72% of suicides among Alaska Native males age 15-24–a group with a suicide rate 14 times the national rate (Alaska Department of Heath & Social Services, 2002). Further, of the 801 deaths attributable in a two-year period to alcohol in Alaska, 36% were Alaska Natives, despite Native people representing only 17% of the state population (Landen, 1996). In contrast to the alarming statistics, scant literature exists on the significant numbers of Alaska Natives who do not abuse alcohol. In addition, one of the last large research studies of alcohol use in Alaska–the Barrow Alcohol Study–ended in significant conflict (Manson, 1989), and enormous suspicion persists that researchers will violate the trust of Native communities. The focus on high rates of alcoholism and its consequences in research and media has contributed to a dominant narrative (Rappaport, 2000) imposed on the Alaska Native community identity that suggests Native people who drink are alcoholic, abuse is inevitable, and sobriety rare. The Alaska Federation of Natives Sobriety Movement is one example of a grassroots movement within the Alaska Native community seeking to counter these perceptions and to foster sobriety. Many Alaska Natives define sobriety to include people who abstain from alcohol or engage in nonproblem alcohol use, as well as those in recovery from alcohol abuse. PA adopted this definition (Hazel & Mohatt, 2001).

We describe two studies; the first qualitative, whose research objective was discovery oriented, and whose specific aim was identification of protective factors in Alaska Native sobriety. Results were used to develop a heuristic model of protective factors, and a measure based on these factors. The research objective of Study 2 was piloting of this measure and initial validation of the instrument's internal structure. Throughout this discussion, we will describe the role of co-researchers in PA, and benefits to the community and co-researchers.

STUDY 1

Participants

For study 1, 37 individuals distributed across sobriety category (life time abstainer, nonproblem drinker, and more than five years abstinence following problem drinking), gender, age, and tribal group, participated in a life history (LH) interview. Another 14 Yup'ik individuals were interviewed using a shorter sobriety pathways focused interview. We over-sampled the Yup'ik cultural group (of 51 interviews, 27 were Yup'ik), as we were designing a Yup'ik culture specific preventative intervention. Participants included 10 lifetime abstainers (5 female/5 male), 19 nonproblem drinkers (9 female/10 male) and 22 individuals abstinent for more than 5 years (9 female/13 male); participant age ranged from 19 to 83 years old, and average age was 49.

Procedures

PA used a participatory action research (PAR) methodology described by Mohatt, Hazel, Allen, Hensel, Stachlerodt, and Fath (in press). Recruitment procedures made extensive use of Alaska Native co-researcher consultants who nominated individuals for participation, with permission of the nominee. Interviewers were Alaska Native co-researchers and university researchers who traveled to participants' communities or, at participants' preference, interviewed at the university. Participants were offered a $25 honorarium, though some declined, considering their story a gift to their communities. Interviews were conducted in a setting of the participant's choice and preferred language; informed consent was obtained prior to the interview. Interviews were recorded digitally, and transcribed verbatim or translated, in cases of indigenous language. Interviewees were given opportunity to review transcripts and/or recordings for accuracy.

A key mechanism of co-researcher involvement was the PA Coordinating Council (PACC), which included Alaska Natives from all regions and major Alaska Native cultural groups. Council members had grassroots activism, personal, or work experience with Native sobriety or alcohol programs. These co-researchers did not function merely as an advisory panel; they engaged in planning and decision-making at each juncture of the research process through ongoing PACC meetings. PA also employed Alaska Native research staff, field research staff, and cultural consultants, all of whom participated in our decision-making. Except in a few cases, these co-researchers did not possess advanced degrees or specialized research training. PA also included several Alaska Native and American Indian students on the university research team.

An important early step in grounding our procedures within Alaska Native culture, and in fostering community acceptance, involved co-researcher involvement in formulation of the research question and selection of methodologies (Hazel & Mohatt, 2001). The co-researcher group decided to focus on sobriety rather than alcoholism, and on cultural and spiritual understandings of this sobriety. In addition, a qualitative approach that honored the narrative and oral traditions of the culture was emphasized as a key component of the research. Co-researchers provided input to the design, structure, and content of the interview procedures (Mohatt, Hazel, et al., in press) and conducted a number of the interviews.

Analysis

Co-researchers engaged with university researchers in a collaborative qualitative data interpretation process. This methodology is described in greater detail in Mohatt, Rasmus, Thomas, Allen, Hazel, Hensel, and PA Team (in review); key co-researcher elements are summarized below. The methodology combined elements of grounded theory analysis (Strauss & Corbin, 1990) with recent methodological advances in team-based (MacQueen, McLellan, Kay, & Milstein, 1998) and consensual analysis (Hill, 1997). Following verbatim transcription and verification with interviewees, procedures included (1) team memoing of transcripts for key themes and initial open coding, (2) open coding of transcripts and coding manual development, (3) formal coding with manual refinement, (4) cultural auditing, (5) generating theories of protective factors through consensual analysis, (6) refining the model of protective factors, then (7) re-assessment of the model, including evaluation of negative cases. Some of the co-researchers trained to work as part of the coding team. *Kappas* ranged from .60 to .81 for 220 lower level formal coding categories, and .90 or above for 25 hierarchical categories. In addition, the PACC met to review interviews, formulate themes, and critique PA research team coding approaches and interpretative work during the cultural auditing phase. Co-researcher collaboration enhanced engagement with participants, facilitating rich, thick description. Credibility of the qualitative findings was also enhanced by co-researcher participation in memoing of narratives, data coding team work, culturally based input to team-based consensual analytic processes, triangulation and critique from multiple co-researcher perspectives, and cultural auditing of the coding and interpretative process.

Results

We identified a set of factors thought to protect youth that both appeared frequently in the narratives of our participants' childhoods and were identified by participants as important to their sobriety. Out of this, a heuristic model of protective factors was developed in collaboration with the PACC; key elements of the model, named in English and Yup'ik, are presented in Figure 1 in developmental chronology, and are described below.

Protective *community characteristics* (CC), *yuut cayarait*, were described by participants to include communities that possessed attributes such as positive adult role models, rites of passage in which one had the opportunity to contribute to the community, limit setting on alcoholic behavior, and provision of safe places for children. One lifetime abstainer described how:

FIGURE 1. Heuristic Model of Protective Factors for Alaska Native Youth

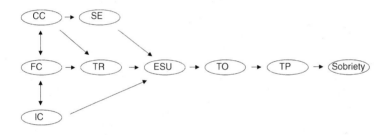

CC (community characteristics) *Nunamta* includes the way the community organizes school, interactions between families, and other important community activities in the life of youth, and enforces alcohol policy and the drinking status of the community.
FC (family characteristics) *Ilaput* includes family functioning in such areas as cohesion, conflict, recreation outlets, moral-spiritual focus, and home organization, and in particular, in the close relationship with at least one parent or caregiver prior to adolescence, who provides praise, social support, safety, good values, and a model of sobriety and giving to others.
IC (individual characteristics) *Yuum Ayuqucia* are communal and personal self-efficacy and *ellangaq*, Yup'ik mindfulness and awareness, or the ability to see connections between one's behavior and its consequences past, present and future.
SE (social environment) *Nunaput* includes role models and social support from extended family, peers, and other adults outside of immediate, nuclear family.
TR (trauma) *Picurlak avillukuk* includes loss/death of loved ones, physical/sexual abuse, and domestic violence. Includes victimization and observation of victimization, perception of trauma and its meaning, and the response to trauma.
ESU (experimental substance use) *Meqerraaryaurtellemni* are early experiences with substances, including alcohol, prior to the establishment of use patterns or abstinence.
TO (thinking it over) *Umyuangcallemni* involves reflecting on one's experience and developing a personal life narrative.
TP (turning point) *Meyirutlemnii* comes out of this reflective process and leads to a decision about how the person will use alcohol.

> We all grew up with five or six different families that you were close with, and that you saw. So we had an extended family. And they, if you were out, or doing something there's always people who knew what you were up to, so if you chose to do something wrong then you knew darn well that your mom and dad were going to know about it when you got home.

Family characteristics (FC), *ilakelriit cayarait*, included important elements of a close relationship with parents. This consisted of a parental teaching role, provision of an environment that was safe and abusive alcoholic behavior was not tolerated, and modeling of sobriety. Expression, often in culture specific ways, of affection and praise, and of specialness of the child, along with the transmission of cultural expectations and values were important. One participant described the force of these factors:

> My mother never, ever drank in her life. And she was always the most steady, the steadying influence on me, and probably my sisters. I would say she's probably the guide through everything. Not only in sobriety, but in our culture, and everything. You know, she was just there, doing things with us.

The protective factor of *individual characteristics* (IC), *yuum ayuqucia*, refers to characteristics of the youth, including wanting to become a role model; giving to others by contributing to the community in both material and less tangible, more interpersonal ways; belief in oneself as someone of value and potential; and awareness of consequences of one's behavior, and of interconnection, described by the Yup'ik as *ellangneq*. One participant described how this awareness suddenly came upon him, dramatically changing his life:

> I was ten years old and I went out to pick berries, I really enjoyed that because I got to get away from everybody and . . . I felt I was being productive. And I just remember picking berries and deciding at the age of ten that I'm not going to drink. I don't want to live that life, I don't want to have the same issues that I grew up with for my own children. I just didn't want that life. (. . .) I can remember that day like it was yesterday. And I have no idea why at such a young age I decided that. I just decided that, and since then it's been hard.

In the qualitative narratives, *individual characteristics* fostered qualities in the youth that included awareness of life goals, and self-efficacy, and a wider sense of communal efficacy. *Family* and *community characteristics* protected children from *trauma exposure* (TR), *akngirneq*, and contributed to a *social environment* (SE), *yuuyaraq*, that included sobriety role models, norms, and peer influences, and support should trauma exposure or crisis occur, particularly during a phase of *experimental substance use* (ESU), *meqerraaryaurtellemni*. A participant described his experience with ESU in this way:

> As I got back to Fairbanks, I started drinking, just having more often. (. . .) But it's one of those things, as soon as I thought that I was building some kind of bad habit, you know, I started doing three beers a night or something, then I just–it's just like something went off, and I said, you know, this is not what I want. And it wasn't like I was getting really high or anything; it's just that I didn't want to get into any kind of rhythm. And so I just pretty much quit for a couple weeks or so and it's really nice that whatever addiction is there is not really there yet.

ESU in most narratives culminated in a period of *thinking over* (TO), *umyuangcallemni*, one's life; all narratives described a *turning point*, (TP) *ayuqucinellemni*, of a conscious decision, typically as an outcome of a reflective process, to not drink or to drink responsibly. Some individuals who engaged in ESU additionally described not liking the taste or the feeling of alcohol, or pointed to episodes of losing control while drinking. Such episodes at times triggered memories of alcohol related trauma from the person's own childhood, initiating TO and TP.

STUDY 2

Participants

Participants included 127 Yup'ik adults living in seven remote villages and a small urban regional center in Southwestern Alaska who completed an extensive survey interview on sobriety and alcohol use, in either Yup'ik or English. Of this sample, 51 reported past or current alcohol use, without having developed an alcohol problem. This group completed the protective factors measure and included 27 females and 24 males, with an average age of 41 years ($SD = 14.2$), and of whom

67% were married and 31% never married; 80% had attended high school, 63% had attended some post secondary education, and 10% had a bachelor's degree. Over 94% reported engaging in subsistence activities, and for 75%, this included hunting and processing large game.

Procedures

The item pool content domain for the protective factors measure was derived from the Study 1 heuristic model. Item content was derived verbatim from statements in the interview transcripts. Items were reviewed and refined by co-researchers on the PA research and Ciuliat Yup'ik

TABLE 1. Internal Structure of the Yup'ik Protective Factors Scale: Principal Component Analysis with Varimax Rotation and Kaiser Normalization

Item	Component			
	1	2	3	4
Things I want for myself, *Wangnun piyumiutenka*				
Saw that drinking leads to violence...	.726	.359	.001	.001
Did not want to lose control of self	.703	.010	.201	.001
Being responsible for other people in the family	.697	.216	.145	.188
Others encouraging you to succeed	.639	.216	.010	.319
Things I want for my family, *Ilamnun piyumiutenka*				
Wanted your kids to have good life	.138	.755	.242	.001
Growing up, wanted to be good role model and respected person	.107	.753	.001	.005
Didn't want to be like those who drank	.187	.588	.221	.210
Embarrassed by drunk family members that drank	.274	.541	.300	.340
Things I want for my body/wellbeing, *Tememnun piyumiutenka*				
Did not like feeling dizzy and high	.001	.172	.851	.003
Did not like feeling embarrassed the next day	.333	.001	.743	.001
Did not like the taste	.256	.332	.688	.002
Things I want for our way of life, *Yuuyaramtenun piyumiutenka*				
You were treated special/unique (inqun)	.119	.001	.001	.762
Want to live up to others' expectations	.007	.155	.293	.749
Was observant and always thinking about what you... (being aware)	.004	.150	−.140	.640

consultant teams (examples are in Table 1). To culturally anchor the instrument, the Ciuliat group, which included Yup'ik cultural experts who did not possess university degrees, Yup'ik human services providers, and Yup'ik university faculty, also reviewed the format and methodology of administration, identifying significant errors of assumptions in many Western research practices regarding how Yup'ik think and operate. Items were then translated into Yup'ik using procedures similar to the committee translation/focus group review procedures advocated by Matýas-Carrelo, Chavez, Negron, Canino, and Aguilar-Hoppe (2003). PA employed interpreters from local communities, and a researcher team member who was bilingual, formatted the survey. In working with translators, co-researchers developed deeper understandings of their indigenous language.

Door to door random sampling for interviewing by strangers was not acceptable to communities in this region. Therefore, we enlisted contacts in each village, typically the village wellness worker (a rural mental health/substance abuse counselor with, or working on a 24-credit certificate degree), to nominate people they believed might be willing to discuss their sobriety and alcohol experiences with our research staff. A PA team flew to a village, usually for most of a week, visited nominees following the wellness worker's introduction, described the study, solicited participation, and obtained informed consent. Participants received a $25 honorarium. The 21-item protective factors survey asked participants to rate how each item "helped you to never have a problem with alcohol," on a five-point likert type scale.[2] As in study 1, data analysis proceeded collaboratively through presentation of results to the PACC, Ciuliat group, and research team, where interpretative perspectives and critiques were offered.

Results

Typically, internal structure of an instrument is identified using factor analysis. In the past, the factor analytic literature has generally recommended large sample sizes (e.g., 10 participants per item) as necessary for stable parameter estimates. This can create serious problems in cultural researcher that often studies groups with small overall population sizes (Okazaki & Sue, 1995) that may live in remote settings. Guadagnoli and Velicer (1988) challenge hard and fast rules for large sample sizes. They present Monte Carlo work demonstrating how variable saturation with factors and number of indicators (items) per factor covaries with sample size to determine the stability of a solution. With loadings approaching .80, solutions were quite stable with samples as small as 50, regardless of the number of indicators, and with smaller numbers of indicators, samples of this size can produce stable solutions with lower loadings.

Prior to analysis, item distributions were reviewed for shape and dispersion, and the 15 best items retained for analyses. Table 1 displays results from a principal components analysis with varimax rotation that yielded a clear structure of four components accounting for 60% of the variance in this small set of indicators. The first protective component–"Things I want for myself, *Wangnun piyumiutenka*"–included personal experiences with loss of control and alcohol related violence, and responsibilities for family. The second component–"Things I want for my family, *Ilamnun piyumiutenka*"–included family and individual characteristics associated with responsibility to children and others. The next component–"Things I want for my body/well-being, *Tememnun piyumiutenka*"–is composed entirely of negative reactions to alcohol's effects, taste, or one's alcohol related behavior. A final factor–"Things I want for our way of life, *Yuuyaramtenun piyumiutenka*"– is quite culture specific, and described appreciation by others (*inquni*), living up to expectations, and personal understanding and practice of *ellangneq*.

Support for the internal validity of this structure can be found in the low intercorrelation of the resulting factor analytically derived subscales, which varied from $r = .09-.50$, and, as shown in Table 2, internal consistencies adequate for research, as well as important gender differences. Women reported higher levels of protective factors on total score, and subscale comparisons, after bonferoni adjustment for multiple comparisons indicated this gender difference occurred in the second protective dimension associated with responsibility to children, role modeling, and not wanting to behave like others who abused alcohol.

DISCUSSION

Alaska Native co-researchers played pivotal roles in PA, a project that successfully formulated a heuristic model to guide prevention interventions, identified protective factors in Alaska Native sobriety, developed a protective factors measure for prevention research, and designed a preventative intervention. The study is notable both for its empirical findings, and because it would not have been possible without the extensive co-researcher involvement. We begin this discussion by de-

TABLE 2. Protective Factors Subscale and Total Score Means, Standard Deviations, and Reliabilities Compared by Gender

Items		α	Gender	M	SD	t(49)
Wangnun piyumiutenka	Scale 1	.69	M	15.4	4.50	−.007
			F	15.4	4.39	
Ilamnun piyumiutenka	Scale 2	.68	M	13.3	4.85	−3.44**
			F	17.4	3.46	
Tememnun piyumiutenka	Scale 3	.73	M	7.4	3.49	−1.83
			F	9.4	4.19	
Yuuyaramtenun piyumiutenka	Scale 4	.59	M	10.5	3.20	−1.03
			F	11.3	2.88	
Total Score		.81	M	49.8	12.62	−2.16*
			F	57.0	11.33	

* $p < .05.$ ** $p < .001.$

scribing how this research links and contributes to existing literature on prevention of American Indian and Alaska Native substance abuse, then describe benefits of the research process to communities and our co-researchers.

Consistent with contemporary theory on adolescent substance abuse (Petraitis, Flay, & Miller, 1995), the resulting PA heuristic model considers triadic influences on community (ultimate), family (distal), and individual (proximal) levels. How these influences function in ethnic minority communities constitute incomplete components within triadic theory (Petraitis, Flay, & Miller, 1995); in particular, little is know regarding protective factors specific to American Indian and Alaska Native cultural contexts (Hawkins, Cummins, & Marlatt, 2004). Though some studies have found limited relation between ethnic identity and substance use among American Indians and Alaska Natives (Bates, Beauvais, & Trimble, 1997), there is strong support for the idea of bicultural competence as decreasing risk (LaFromboise, Coleman, & Gerton, 1993). Within the realm of bicultural competence, this study is significant in its identification of culture specific elements of bicultural competence in Yup'ik Alaska Natives, on the level of the community, family, and individual, described as protective from alcohol abuse by Alaska Natives. The protective factors measure developed out of the research taps a more complex construct, and its various subscales include items that range from predispositional factors in the individual such as taste aversion, to competencies such as the sense of responsibility to others and of being aware. These elements identified in the research provide important foci and measurable outcomes for substance abuse prevention interventions in Alaska Native communities, and the measure provides an individual level assessment tool.

Level of co-researcher involvement was extensive and significant throughout the research process, from formulation of the research question and selection of the methodology, to data collection, analysis, and interpretation. The PACC and Ciuliat participated in planning and decision-making while Alaska Native and American Indian student and co-researcher staff worked alongside university researchers. Co-researchers facilitated the data collection process; they were often familiar with the communities, personally knew several residents, and could provide introductions to community leaders. Co-researcher staff were also typically more successful in recruiting research participants, as they spoke the language and lent legitimacy to project's claims that the research was being conducted collaboratively with Alaska Natives. In the remaining sections of this article, we describe several benefits to Alaska Native communities that resulted from the co-researcher involvement, as well as several benefits to the co-researchers themselves. We also describe future areas of research for co-researcher involvement in PAR methodologies, and draw some conclusions regarding this type of work in culturally distinct communities.

Benefits to the Community

From the very beginning, the PACC, our co-researchers, insisted on products from research that could be shared with communities to help prevent alcohol abuse and help people who are struggling find and maintain their sobriety path. One immediate and tangible outcome of the project thus far is the creation of an innovative multimedia program (CD-ROM format) on Alaska Native sobriety, with a companion booklet of life history sketches of selected participants (People Awakening Project, 2003) authored to appeal to youth. The CD-ROM provides pictures, voice, and narratives of Alaska Natives who became sober or never had a drinking problem, a graphic arts presentation of the PA heuristic model, and point and click search capabilities embedded in the graphics in this model hyperlinked to digital recordings of oral narratives on the topic. These two tools serve as the basis for the multi-level preventive intervention. The narrative format fits the face-to-face, oral culture, and can contribute to private, individual exploration congruent with Alaska Native learning styles (Lipka, Mohatt, & Ciulistet Group, 1998).

A second benefit to communities was a culturally grounded prevention intervention to enhance community, family, and individual protective factors identified by PA among rural Yup'ik youth, designed by the co-researchers with university researchers using key elements of a tribal participatory methods process (Fisher & Ball, 2002). The PA theoretical model and findings are used to support the intervention's culture specific elements in grant funding applications. If the intervention proves effective, co-researcher involvement will have been central in PA's ability to give back to the community. Implementation of the intervention will make extensive use of a local Alaska Native staff that does not possess advanced professional degrees, and outcome research to demonstrate the hypothesized efficacy of the intervention will use current PA co-researchers as PACC members, consultants, translators, and research staff. A key component of evaluation of the proposed intervention, in addition to effectiveness, is an ethnographic process evaluation to document implementation, benefits to co-researchers/interventionists, and benefits to the community. We also anticipate the evaluation will elucidate important ways in which preventative interventions must be grounded in cultural factors for successful implementation in Alaska Native communities.

Third, the work of the PA co-researchers has been instrumental in providing models for increased local control of the research process for indigenous communities. We hope that these models and the experience gained, furthers community understanding of how research skills and findings from research can enhance self-determination in Native communities, regarding social programs and social policy. In one small way, we hope the efforts of PA contribute to changes in the dominant narrative regarding alcohol and Alaska Natives.

Benefits to the Co-Researchers

Co-researchers benefited from the training and experience in interviewing. One co-researcher, who had struggled with alcohol abuse, described how hearing stories of others helped him to understand his own sobriety process. He also felt he benefited when he could listen and offer others support. Several changes were noted in the co-researcher group. Through a process somewhat akin to on the job training, co-researchers developed enhanced research sophistication. Co-researchers took on increasingly complex tasks, and offered increasingly probing critiques regarding methodology, analyses, and interpretation. One co-researcher enrolled in graduate school through the process. The PACC, Ciuliat group, and PA staff now comprise a cadre of Alaska Native people with considerable research sophistication for future studies. Enhancement of interest in research to identify solutions to problems is also evident in the frequent requests PA has received for presentations to key Alaska Native groups. The regional Alaska Native health corporation instrumental in PA's access to communities, followed the work closely and now wishes to move forward with intervention.

Benefits to the University Researchers

Though benefits to the community and co-researchers are the focus of this special volume, it would be misleading to characterize the PA process as one-way. The university researchers also benefited from co-researcher involvement. Co-researchers educated them regarding appropriate methods of seeking invitation into communities, research procedures acceptable to Native communities, and more culturally grounded interpretations of the PA data. They also enhanced the credibility and validity of the research findings from Native communities by providing university researchers an enhanced, deeper understanding of the data.

Directions for Future Research

PAR methodology and use of Alaska Native co-researchers can continue to provide beneficial outcomes in several future areas for research that build on these study findings. These include work to (1) develop similar emically derived measures of culture specific protective strategies for the four other Alaska Native cultural groups, (2) test the culture specific preventative intervention developed for youth in the Yup'ik region, (3) develop and test culture specific preventative interventions with the four other Alaska Native cultural groups, (4) understand how these protective factors can be applied in treatment, and particularly in relapse prevention, and (5) conduct more thorough and systematic assessments of the impact of the PAR approach on the research participants, co-researchers, and communities. In particular, little is known on how these methods are perceived, experienced, and impact communities. There has been especially limited attention to how nondominant culturally distinct communities may view research and its outcomes in quite different ways than researchers. This study shares this limitation with much of the PAR literature in lacking data based assessment of impact. An explicitly stated outcome of PAR methods is a process of empowerment, or *conscientization* (Freire, 1970). Future studies should directly assess for this and other outcomes among co-researchers and communities. However, in making these recommendations, we wish to also highlight the paramount importance of co-researcher involvement in the formulation of these and other research questions in ways that address local concerns and best serve their communities.

CONCLUSIONS

In many ways, this research on protective factors was about the *"tools to understand"* that are resident and can only be found in Native community members themselves. The Alaska Native co-researchers brought several skills with them to the PA process, not the least of which was insider knowledge regarding communities. In addition to development of the research capacity of Alaska Native communities and a preventative intervention, PA's utilization of co-researchers has provided a model for research in Alaska Native communities that enhances community control of the research process. Co-researcher involvement and the PAR approach brought about a different type of research relationship than typically found in alcohol research, and a research setting that was more culturally competent, in that it was in greater accord with Native values. What is also significant about PA is that its formulation of protective factors emerged from an Alaska Native context, through significant involvement of individuals whose daily lives were grounded in this cultural context, rather than that of professional researchers. This moves us closer to an *emic* (Berry, 1969) understanding of protective factors, with important implications for research methodologies in ethnic minority communities and a multicultural society. In the end, this may prove the greatest benefit to communities and co-researchers that comes out of PA and efforts similar to it.

NOTES

1. The People Awakening Project (PA) team includes the PA Coordinating Council, who are: Robert Charlie, Samuel Demientieff, Mary Miller, Don Mironov, Valerie Naquin, Elizabeth "Cookie" Rose, David Sam, Judy Simeonoff, Doreen Simmonds,

Elvina Turner, Annie Wassilie and George Charles; the Ciuliat Group/the PA Yup'ik Advisory Council and Translation Group, who are: Eliza Orr, Anna Jacobson, Marty Hintz, Lorita Clough, Annie Wasuli, and Walkie Charles; the PA project staff, who are: Mary Stachelrodt, Chase Hensel, Alice Atuk, Dante Foster; and the following individuals: Dolores Scoville, Carol Yakish, Caroline Brown, David Charles, Sue Charles, Kelly McGuire and Jamie Mohatt.

2. Several participants rated the likert type items using a graphically-based tool with a sliding mechanism that was developed by M. Stachelrodt of the PA research team based on suggestions from W. Charles of the Ciuliat Group.

REFERENCES

Alaska Department of Health & Social Services [DHSS]. (2002). *Healthy Alaskans 2010: Targets and strategies for improved health. Volume 1: Targets for improved health.* Juneau: Alaska Department of Health and Social Services. Division of Public Health.

Bates, S. C., Beauvais, F., & Trimble, J. E. (1997). American Indian adolescent alcohol involvement and ethnic identification. *Substance Use and Misuse, 32,* 2013-2031.

Berry, J.W. (1969). On cross-cultural comparability. *International Journal of Psychology, 4,* 119-128.

Chesler, M. A. (1991). Participatory Action Research with self-help groups: An alternative paradigm for inquiry and action. *American Journal of Community Psychology, 19,* 757-768.

Fisher, P. A. & Ball, T. J. (2002). The Indian Family Wellness Project: An application of the tribal participatory research model. *Prevention Science, 3,* 235-240.

Freire, P. (1970). *Pedagogy of the oppressed.* New York: Continuum Publishing Co.

Guadagnoli, E. & Velicer, W. F. (1988). Relation of sample size to the stability of component patterns. *Psychological Bulletin, 103,* 265-275.

Hawkins, E. H., Cummins, L. H., and Marlatt, G. A. (2004). Preventing substance abuse in American Indian and Alaska Native youth: Promising strategies for healthier communities. *Psychological Bulletin, 130,* 304-323.

Hazel, K. L. & Mohatt, G. V. (2001). Cultural and spiritual coping in sobriety: Informing substance abuse prevention for Alaska Native communities. *Journal of Community Psychology, 29,* 541-562.

Hill, C. E., Thompson, B. J., & Williams, E. N. (1997). A guide to conducting consensual qualitative research. *The Counseling Psychologist. 25,* 517-572.

LaFromboise, T. D., Coleman, H. L. K., & Gerton, J. (1993). Psychological impact of biculturalism: Evidence and theory. *Psychological Bulletin, 114,* 395-412.

Landen, M. G. (1996). Alcohol related mortality in Alaska: 1992-1994. *State of Alaska Epidemiology Bulletin, 6.* Anchorage: Department of Health and Social Services, Division of Public Health, Section of Epidemiology.

Lipka, J., Mohatt, G.V., & Ciulistet (1998). *Transforming school: Yup'ik case examples.* Garden City: Erlbaum Press.

MacQueen, K. M., McLellan, E., Kay, K., & Milstein, B. (1998). Codebook development for team-based qualitative analysis. *Cultural Anthropology Methods, 10,* 31-36.

Manson, S. M. (1989). Barrow alcohol study: Emphasis on its ethical and procedural aspects. [Special Issue]. *American Indian and Alaska Native Mental Health Research, 2*, 5-6.

Matýas-Carrelo, L. E., Chavez, L. M., Negron, G., Canino, G., Aguilar-Hoppe, S. (2003). The Spanish translation and cultural adaptation of five mental health measures. *Culture, Medicine and Psychiatry 27*, 291–313.

Mohatt, G. V., Rasmus, S. M., Thomas, L. Allen, J., Hazel, K., Hensel, C., & PA Team. (in review). *Tied Together Like a Woven Hat: Protective Pathways to Sobriety For Alaska Natives*. Fairbanks AK: University of Alaska Fairbanks.

Mohatt, G.V., Hazel, K., Allen, J., Hensel, C., Stachlerodt, M., & Fath, R. (in press). Unheard Alaska: Participatory Action Research on Sobriety with Alaska Natives. *American Journal of Community Psychology*.

Okazaki, S. & Sue, S. (1995). Methodological issues in assessment research with ethnic minorities. *Psychological Assessment, 7*, 367-375.

People Awakening Project. (2003). *"My Way to Myself": Alaska Native pathways toward sobriety*. [CD-ROM]. C. Hensel, S.M. Rasmus, G.V. Mohatt, & PA Team, (Eds.). Psychology Department and Rasmuson Library, Project Jukebox: University of Alaska Fairbanks.

Petraitis, J., Flay, B. R. & Miller, T. Q. (1995). Reviewing theories of adolescent substance abuse: Organizing pieces of the puzzle. *Psychological Bulletin, 117*, 67-86.

Rappaport, J. (2000). Community narratives: Tales of terror and joy. *American Journal of Community Psychology, 28*, 1-24.

Rutter, M. (2000). Resilience reconsidered: Conceptual considerations, empirical findings, and policy implications. In J. P. Shonkoff & S. J. Meisels, (Eds.), *Handbook of early childhood intervention* (2nd ed.). New York: Cambridge University Press.

Strauss, A., & Corbin, J. (1990). *Basics of qualitative research: Grounded theory procedures and techniques*. Newbury Park, CA: Sage Publications.

White, G. W., Nary, D. E., Froehlich, A. K. (2001). Consumers as collaborators in research and action, *Journal of Prevention and Intervention in the Community, 21*, 15-35.

An Evaluation of the Effects
of Neighborhood Mobilization
on Community Problems

Patrick G. Donnelly
Charles E. Kimble

University of Dayton

SUMMARY. This research examines the outcomes of actions taken by members of a residential neighborhood association to revitalize a neighborhood and to make it a safer and more secure place to live. This urban neighborhood association initiated a major planning process in cooperation with city officials. Residents overwhelmingly adopted the plan that included the creation of mini-neighborhoods with a series of gates to moderate traffic flow, increase neighborliness, and reduce crime. An analysis of official data from police crime reports shows that crime was significantly reduced in the neighborhood after the street changes. This reduction in crime was maintained even five years later. Telephone in-

Address correspondence to: Patrick G. Donnelly, Department of Sociology, Anthropology and Social Work, University of Dayton, Dayton, OH 45469-1442 (E-mail: donnelly@udayton.edu).

The authors wish to thank Roger Reeb and David Biers for their helpful comments on an earlier version of this paper. They also thank the Dayton Police Department for providing the police crime data used in this paper. All analysis and interpretations are the responsibility of the authors.

This research was supported in part by the City of Dayton and the University of Dayton Summer Fellowship Program.

[Haworth co-indexing entry note]: "An Evaluation of the Effects of Neighborhood Mobilization on Community Problems." Donnelly, Patrick G. and Charles E. Kimble. Co-published simultaneously in *Journal of Prevention & Intervention in the Community* (The Haworth Press, Inc.) Vol. 32, No. 1/2, 2006, pp. 61-80; and: *Community Action Research: Benefits to Community Members and Service Providers* (ed: Roger N. Reeb) The Haworth Press, Inc., 2006, pp. 61-80. Single or multiple copies of this article are available for a fee from The Haworth Document Delivery Service [1-800-HAWORTH, 9:00 a.m. - 5:00 p.m. (EST). E-mail address: docdelivery@haworthpress.com].

terviews with neighborhood residents indicated that they perceived re-
ductions in traffic, crime, noise and drug offenses for at least five years
after the changes. Even though neighborhood cohesion did not increase,
it appears that the actions instigated and promoted by neighborhood association members enhanced the quality of life for neighborhood residents. *[Article copies available for a fee from The Haworth Document Delivery
Service: 1-800-HAWORTH. E-mail address: <docdelivery@haworthpress.com>
Website: <http://www.HaworthPress.com> © 2006 by The Haworth Press, Inc.
All rights reserved.]*

KEYWORDS. Neighborhood associations, civic involvement, community crime prevention, resident participation, community problems

From the time of Alexis de Tocqueville, social scientists have noted
the extent to which Americans participate in a wide range of voluntary
associations "of a thousand kinds" (de Tocqueville, 1969, p. 517). The
associations, ranging from school and church groups to service and fra-
ternal organizations, from labor unions to political groups, were viewed
as indispensable to the functioning of the American democratic system
organizations. In recent years, there has been widespread discussion
about the extent, direction, and nature of civic involvement, and a
broader discussion about the importance of such involvement in the
context of a global society.

Robert Putnam's (1995) concept of "bowling alone" suggests that
civic involvement has declined in recent years. Using data from membership reports, polls, and voting records, he argues that Americans to-
day are much less civic-minded than even a generation earlier. While
other authors challenge some of the data cited by Putnam, there is agreement that changes in families, corporations, government, and in communities themselves have created new situations affecting individuals'
participation in community life. Dual career parents or single parents,
and job relocations or extended workweeks are just a few examples of
changes that affect individuals' participation in the traditional civic organizations. But many Americans want to remain engaged in the community and deliberately search for community connections, although
considerably looser, more flexible, ad hoc connections than those of
previous generations (Bellah, Madsen, Sullivan, Swidler & Tipton,
1985; Wuthnow, 2002).

In general, civic involvement frequently occurs in voluntary associations that serve a number of purposes: they mediate between citizens

and larger structures of the state and market; they temper the negative social tendencies associated with state and market; and they inculcate democratic values and habits (Eberly, 2000). They provide a voice and an opportunity for individuals and groups to shape the conditions that affect their lives. This article examines the role of citizens in a type of community organization commonly found in urban areas, the neighborhood association (NA). In particular, it will analyze empirical data to assess the efficacy of the efforts of these volunteer members to implement a strategic plan for the neighborhood. The goal of the plan was to stabilize this racially and economically diverse neighborhood by reducing a variety of problems and enhancing the sense of community within the neighborhood.

While neighborhood organizations may vary in their focus, organization, size and other aspects, they all are civic organizations oriented toward maintaining or improving the quality of life in a geographically delimited area (Logan & Rabrenovic, 1990). To accomplish this, NAs develop and offer a range of community services for neighborhood residents. They may offer social and recreational activities; they help create a sense of community by bringing residents together; they serve as a vehicle to share information about what is going on in the neighborhood; they are a conduit of information between residents and city government; they direct attention and coordinate responses to neighborhood concerns including housing, traffic and crime; and, more recently, they have become more involved in instrumental political activities to enhance the quality of life within communities. NAs frequently focus on neighborhood issues that may reflect changes in the external environment. Changes in regional housing markets may pressure cities to examine zoning changes; regional demographic changes may affect neighborhoods' poverty, unemployment and crime rates; broader political factors may raise issues concerning landfill or environmental hazards for communities. Active NAs respond to these changes in order to minimize the negative consequences that they may have on their communities.

Considerable research has been done on various types of neighborhood organizations. Rabrenovic (1996) found a number of successful efforts to stabilize neighborhoods, address neighborhood problems, and promote quality of life issues. The more successful efforts appear to occur when neighborhood groups effectively mobilize their residents and when local governments allow the participation of neighborhood groups in the decision-making process. Effective resident mobilization is easier in cohesive and homogenous communities than in fragmented and diverse communities. Efforts at mobilizing racially and economically diverse communities may be less successful because of the difficulty of gaining a common set of goals and strategies that address the perceived needs of the different groups. Successful neighborhood efforts are also related to local governments with resources and an openness to collaboration with community groups. Rabrenovic suggests that these are less likely to be found in older industrial-based cites than in more service-based cities.

Efforts by NAs to enhance neighborhoods may be seen as clear examples of community service projects. They offer community programs or services to residents and offer a collective voice in dealing with external organizations and pressures. As with many community service efforts, there is an element of self-interest in the work of NAs. Residents may engage in various projects because it improves the quality of life for themselves and their families and also because it maintains their own property values. At times, NAs may be divided by differences in goals with some groups primarily focused on protecting their economic investment in their homes while others may place a higher priority on neighborhood quality of life (Rabrenovic, 1996). This paper describes a major effort of a NA to enhance the positive features of one neighborhood including its sense of community and to reduce negative features including crime. Following a general description of the neighborhood and the development of the strategic plan, the results of Study 1, which focused on crime data from the city police department, and Study 2, which focused on survey data obtained by residents, will be presented.

BACKGROUND

Brief Description of the Neighborhood

The Five Oaks neighborhood is an older, inner-ring city neighborhood located about one mile north of the downtown area of Dayton, Ohio, a city with a shrinking population that totaled 165,000 in 2000. Built mostly during the 1920s to house working and middle income residents, the Five Oaks neighborhood is basically laid out in a traditional grid pattern with about 10 east-west and 10 north-south streets. It is bordered by two major north-south streets that carry many daily commuters to and from downtown. It has a population of just under 5,000 residents and a few commercial enterprises.

Like many inner-ring neighborhoods, Five Oaks was undergoing a number of demographic changes in recent decades. In 1970, the population of the neighborhood was 97% white and 3% minority. By 1990, Five Oaks was 52% white and 46% African-American. The economic status of the neighborhood changed as evidenced by rising poverty rates and declining homeownership rates. When the crack epidemic arrived in Dayton in the late 1980s, it hit Five Oaks and surrounding neighborhoods hard. Drug houses were established in these areas, facilitated by the changing housing market and the ease of access to the neighborhood from major streets and highways. There was also an increase in other types of crimes including robberies and burglaries. Other signs of disorder, such as prostitution and speeding cars, may appear to be less serious but disheartened many residents who felt that they were losing control of the neighborhood (Donnelly & Majka, 1998).

The Strategic Plan

In 1990 the neighborhood association began to organize a major effort to address the problems and promote greater resident participation in the neighborhood. The Five Oaks Neighborhood Improvement Association (FONIA) had been in existence since the late 1970s and was one of the more active NAs in the city. While much of its early efforts focused on housing issues, it also worked on broader community building programs that included social and recreational programs for youth and adults. It effectively lobbied city hall for programs that improved services to neighborhood residents. FONIA held monthly neighborhood meetings and was led by a board of volunteers elected by residents. Most monthly meetings drew a few dozen residents but many more people would attend and participate in the various programs and activities sponsored by FONIA. Periodically, FONIA would form committees to address various issues and would recruit residents to participate.

To address the problems affecting Five Oaks in the early 1990s, FONIA worked with the city to develop a stabilization plan for one of the few racially and economically diverse neighborhoods in the city. The role of FONIA in this case must be understood in light of the City of Dayton's national reputation for encouraging citizen participation in public affairs. A 1993 book, *The Rebirth of Urban Democracy*, published by the Brookings Institute, cited Dayton as one of five U.S. cities that has "transformed the political life of their communities" by establishing a system of neighborhood organizations to promote citizen participation in public decision-making (Berry, Portnoy & Thompson,

1993). The system gave neighborhood groups "substantial authority over decisions that affect the quality of life in their communities, and they facilitate participation of rank-and-file citizens in face-to-face settings" (p. 283). A writer for *Governing*, a magazine for city officials and planners, refers to Dayton as "the state of the art in citizen participation." It has "remarkably assertive neighborhoods and neighborhood activists, accustomed to taking matters in hands and to getting a response from department heads and city officials" (Gurwitt, 1992, p. 48).

Resident Participation in the Plan

Yet, even in this city with a renowned reputation for volunteer efforts and activism, the plan created by FONIA was distinctive. The City Manager of Dayton said that "FONIA prepared the most elaborate citizen participation mechanism this City has known" (Helwig, 1993). This elaborate process emerged after members of FONIA met with key city officials several times in the summer of 1991. FONIA members discussed the serious drug and crime problems confronting residents and their concern that there would be further middle class flight from the neighborhood. City officials pointed to the difficulties they faced in making "good drug buys" that allowed them to gather the evidence needed to convict the drug dealers. FONIA members argued that if action was not taken soon, many homes would go up for sale and that the racial and economic diversity of the neighborhood would be lost.

The meetings led to a mutual agreement: the city would take immediate action on the drug activity in Five Oaks and FONIA would review and update its 1985 strategic plan. The city quickly carried through on its commitment. The police conducted drug raids and made numerous arrests in Five Oaks and the surrounding neighborhoods. But before they did, they notified local media of their plans so that the raids would be widely publicized. The raids were the lead story on the late night news and in the morning paper, and were covered by the media over the next few days. This was done to restore confidence among residents that the city was making a serious effort to confront the problems.

FONIA created a Strategic Plan Committee that consisted of ten residents, a city planner, and representatives of the five key institutions in the neighborhood: three churches, one school, and a hospital. The residents included both elected FONIA leaders as well as other residents who expressed a willingness to participate. The committee began work in December 1991 and identified several major issues: traffic, crime and safety, housing, sense of community, and public relations. The FONIA

Plan Committee invited residents to serve on the various subgroups that were created to address each of the major issues.

The committee was informed that the Dayton Police Department had invited a nationally recognized urban planner, Oscar Newman, to visit Dayton to discuss ways of shaping the physical environment to reduce crime. Newman's concept of defensible space had been implemented in a number of other American cities (Newman, 1972, 1995). After hearing Newman's presentation, the committee asked the city to invite Newman to propose a plan for Five Oaks. Newman toured Five Oaks with city officials and residents and then met with members of the Strategic Plan Committee. The committee suggested ways to adapt Newman's concept to Five Oaks and made several changes in his initial designs.

Recognizing that the defensible space plan, which involved closing streets and alleys, would require widespread resident participation and consensus, the committee developed a plan to involve as many residents as possible. The committee recruited over 40 volunteers from each section of the neighborhood to "walk n' talk" the neighborhood. Many volunteers had previously been involved in various FONIA-sponsored activities. Over a 10-day period, the volunteers went to all of the 1,800 housing units to talk with residents, drop off a flyer, and invite them to the FONIA meeting. FONIA mailed a postcard to every housing unit announcing the meeting. In addition, the regular monthly FONIA newsletter was hand-delivered to every household. Over 400 people attended the March meeting to hear the presentations about the plan by FONIA members, Newman, and city officials. Numerous questions, challenges, and suggestions were raised by those in attendance. After three hours, a straw poll taken on whether the committee should continue refining the plan was overwhelmingly approved (Five Oaks Neighborhood Improvement Association, 1993).

FONIA developed a plan to hold a series of ten mini-neighborhood meetings. Captains were selected to advertise and lead these smaller gatherings where residents could examine and discuss what the plan would mean for their section of the neighborhood. Again, volunteers walked n' talked every household to invite residents to attend. Attendance at the meetings ranged from a dozen in two areas to over 75 in others. A few of the mini-neighborhoods had second or third meetings to refine the plan or work out disagreements. At the conclusion of these meetings, residents were allowed to vote on the plan. Meanwhile, committee members met with representatives of various city departments including fire, police, and waste collection to discuss the plan. The local bus company, emergency medical services, and local institutions were also consulted.

The April FONIA meeting drew over 300 residents to hear reports from the mini-neighborhood captains, city officials, and committee members. Several issues were raised about the street closures that dealt with emergency response time, the cost of the project, and the inconveniences that would be created. Police and fire officials as well as committee members responded to the issues that were raised. At the end of the meeting, residents were asked to vote on the final plan. When all 600 votes were tallied, the plan passed 93%-7%.

FONIA leaders estimate that well over 5,000 hours of volunteer labor went into the project (Five Oaks Neighborhood Improvement Association, 1993). This number includes residents' time in the working sessions on the committee and FONIA, the walk n' talk efforts, and the meetings with various local groups. Over 40 meetings were held to develop the plan. These hours do not include residents' attendance at the FONIA meetings. Including all the hours that residents spent at neighborhood meetings would clearly drive the total hours over 10,000. For its efforts in developing the plan, FONIA received recognition by the national organization, Neighborhoods, USA as 1993 Neighborhood of the Year.

The 20 page Five Oaks Neighborhood Stabilization Plan contained six elements: the defensible space plan, a home ownership program, social and recreational programming, housing code enforcement, coordination of community-based policing, and a revised organizational structure for FONIA (Five Oaks Neighborhood Improvement Association and the City of Dayton, 1993). The defensible space plan led to the closing of 36 streets at one end of the block with gates as well as the closing of 26 alleys. The gates prevent vehicular traffic but permit pedestrians or bicycle traffic on the open sidewalks. The home ownership plan provided assistance for first time homebuyers in Five Oaks. FONIA established or maintained a number of recreational programs for youth. An on-site office was established for the community-based police officer and regular communication with the officer was maintained by FONIA. The FONIA constitution was amended to require area-wide elections, as opposed to neighborhood-wide elections, to ensure that all smaller areas within the neighborhood were represented on the board. While the City of Dayton invested considerable time and over $450,000 in the plan (Helwig, 1993), and while professional urban planners were involved in its development, it is clear that many Five Oaks residents viewed it as their own plan. Residents had invested so much personal time and effort in developing the plan, that they took ownership of the plan (Donnelly & Majka, 1998).

STUDY 1

Method

In order to evaluate the outcomes of the Five Oaks stabilization plan for the neighborhood and its residents, two types of data were collected. In Study 1, crime data collected by the city police department before and after the plan was implemented is used to examine the effects of the plan. Crime data for Five Oaks, surrounding neighborhoods, and for the City of Dayton as a whole for the period from 1990 through 1997 are examined to determine the changes in crime over time. Following up on a previous study (Donnelly & Kimble, 1997), crime data are first analyzed for 1992 and 1993, the periods immediately preceding and following the implementation of the plan. Then the data are analyzed for a longer period from 1990 to 1997 to determine any long-range effects of the plan. Changes in the number of crimes in Five Oaks are compared with changes in crime in surrounding neighborhoods and in the City of Dayton as a whole. The surrounding neighborhoods are similar to Five Oaks in many ways. While the population of Five Oaks was 46% African American in 1990, the surrounding neighborhoods were 48% African American. Rates of homeownership and vacant housing units were 35% and 15% in Five Oaks and 31% and 16% respectively in the adjacent areas. The crime data for surrounding neighborhoods and for the city as a whole serve as a comparison group. Data on total crimes, serious violent crimes, and other types of offenses in these areas are examined.

Results and Discussion

The entire stabilization plan was approved, and much of it implemented in late 1992. To determine the effects of the plan on the neighborhood and its residents, this analysis compares data from 1992 and before with data from 1993 and later. Table 1 shows the increase in crime in Five Oaks from 1991 to 1992 that, in part, precipitated that plan. It also shows the significant decreases in crime immediately following implementation of the plan. Total criminal offenses dropped from 1,161 in 1992 to 888 in 1993, a decrease of 24%. The number of violent crimes reported in Five Oaks declined 40% immediately after the plan was implemented. There was also a 22% decline in other offenses from their high totals in 1992.

TABLE 1. Crime in Five Oaks, 1990-1997

Crime	1990	1991	1992	1993	1994	1995	1996	1997
Homicide	2	2	1	1	1	2	2	0
Rape	5	6	6	14	6	9	9	2
Robbery	33	40	67	35	47	42	23	31
Aggravated Assault	20	40	45	21	19	20	12	10
Sub-Total Violent Crime	60	88	119	71	73	73	46	43
Other Assaults	207	207	225	200	212	217	142	143
Burglary	118	168	181	110	103	111	117	104
Larceny	209	222	251	189	182	237	196	186
Auto Theft	83	58	61	52	62	96	76	61
Arson	8	7	12	2	5	4	9	5
Vandalism	194	138	188	148	167	196	130	118
Carrying Concealed Weapon	3	7	6	9	4	3	8	4
Prostitution	10	22	14	8	3	6	9	4
Narcotics	14	23	13	11	20	19	41	25
Intoxication	2	0	7	0	0	2	6	1
Miscellaneous (all other offenses)	65	78	84	88	79	104	90	89
Sub-total non-Violent Crime	913	930	1,042	817	837	994	824	740
GRAND TOTAL	973	1,018	1,161	888	910	1,067	870	783

Table 2 shows that crime also declined in the adjoining neighborhoods and in the city as a whole between 1992 and 1993. But the significant declines in crime in Five Oaks are greater than the declines in adjoining neighborhoods and in the whole city. The 24% drop in total crimes in Five Oaks from 1992 to 1993 (χ^2 (1) = 36.37, $p < .0001$) is much greater than the 3% drop in surrounding areas (χ^2 (1) = 9.64, $p < .002$) and the almost imperceptible drop in crime in the city (χ^2 (1) = 0.00, $p = .96$).

TABLE 2. Crime in Five Oaks Neighborhood, Nearby Neighborhoods, and City of Dayton, 1990-1997

Areas	1990	1991	1992	1993	1994	1995	1996	1997
Five Oaks								
Total Crime	973	1,018	1,161	888	910	1,067	870	766
Violent	60	88	119	71	73	73	46	43
Other	913	924	1,042	817	837	994	824	723
Nearby								
Total Crime	3,659	3,986	4,088	3,950	3,473	3,579	3,079	2,913
Violent	376	390	430	316	289	289	192	167
Other	3,283	3,596	3,658	3,634	3,192	3,290	2,887	2,746
Dayton								
Total Crime	45,219	44,390	41,782	41,767	37,598	41,160	39,668	37,281
Violent	3,257	3,679	3,523	3,139	2,639	2,539	2,100	2,161
Other	41,962	40,611	38,259	38,628	34,959	38,621	37,568	35,120

The number of serious violent crimes committed in Five Oaks in the year after the plan was implemented declined by 40%, χ^2 (1) = 12.13, $p <$ .0001, compared to the 26% decline in nearby neighborhoods, χ^2 (1) = 17.42, $p < $ .00001, and the 11% decline in the city, χ^2 (1) = 22.13, $p <$ .00001. The Chi Square for the decline in violent crimes in Five Oaks is lower than that in nearby neighborhoods and the city due to the low absolute number of violent crime in Five Oaks. Other crimes also declined more in Five Oaks (21.6%) than in the nearby neighborhoods (0.6%) and in the City of Dayton (1% increase) in the first year. The change in the number of other offenses in Five Oaks from 1992 to 1993 was significant, χ^2 (1) = 27.23, $p < $ .00001 while the changes in the two comparison areas were not significant.

A comparison of the mean number of offenses in pre-plan years (1990-1992) with the mean in the post-plan years (1993-1997) was undertaken to see if the changes in crime endured over time. When we compared the pre-plan and post-plan averages in Five Oaks, we found a significant 14.2% reduction in total crimes (χ^2 (1) = 11.39, $p < $ .001); a 31.5% reduction in serious violent crimes (χ^2 (1) = 5.23, $p < $ .025); and a 12.6% reduction in other crimes (χ^2 (1) = 8.14, $p < $ .005) since the implementation of the plan. Overall, there was a lasting reduction in crime in Five Oaks following the implementation of the plan.

For the longer period, the decline in total crime in Five Oaks (33%) was greater than the decline in the surrounding areas (30%) and the city

(8%). However, 2 × 2 chi square analyses showed that there were no significant differences between the long-term decline in Five Oaks and the declines of the nearby neighborhoods or the city for total, violent, or other crimes. While there were greater decreases in crime in Five Oaks in the first year after the changes than in the surrounding areas and in the city, there were not statistically significant differences between the changes in crime in Five Oaks and the other areas over the entire five post-change years. It should be noted that the decreases in crime in the nearby neighborhoods and the city that occurred over time may have been influenced somewhat by the Five Oaks changes. For instance, some of the surrounding neighborhoods copied some of the ideas used by FONIA and changed their traffic patterns by creating one-way streets, closed streets, and installing speed bumps.

One initial concern with the plan was that it would merely displace the crime from Five Oaks to surrounding neighborhoods. It is not possible in this research to determine if any of the criminal activity or any of the criminals who would have committed their offenses in Five Oaks simply moved to other areas. However, the fact that crime went down so precipitously in Five Oaks and that it also went down in surrounding neighborhoods and the city as a whole suggests that crime displacement did not occur to any significant degree.

STUDY 2

Police data on crime provide a limited, and potentially biased view of crime. These data depend on residents reporting an offense to the police and the police officer filing of a report. Most crimes that are committed are not reported to the police because victims do not feel the offense is important enough or because they believe that police would not be able to do anything about it (Bureau of Justice Statistics, 2003). Other offenses are not reported because residents do not want to get involved.

Method

To offset the problem noted above, Study 2 involved conducting interviews with Five Oaks residents to determine their perceptions of safety and crime, as well as other aspects of the neighborhood. These telephone interviews were conducted at three different times, once immediately prior to the implementation of the plan, once immediately after the implementation, and again five years later. Randomly selected telephone numbers in the neighborhood were drawn each year using the Criss-Cross Directory. This method excludes from the sample households with no phones and those with unlisted numbers. The interviews were conducted by trained students supervised by the authors through a university social science research center. Approximately 180 completed interviews were used in each survey. Table 3 presents a description of the three samples.

Results and Discussion

Residents were asked a series of questions about their perceptions of neighborhood conditions, including questions related to the seriousness of various types of crimes. Average seriousness ratings were computed

TABLE 3. Demographic Characteristics of Respondents in Percent

		1992	1993	1998
Gender	Male	35	43	41
	Female	65	57	59
Age	18-34	28	25	24
	35-59	44	42	56
	60 +	28	33	21
Highest Grade Completed	12	37	40	29
	15	27	27	29
	16 +	35	33	42
Marital Status	Single	55	48	50
	Married	45	52	50
Number of Children in Household	0	56	56	54
	1-2	27	29	30
	3 +	17	15	16
Race	White	74	74	72
	Black	24	24	22
	Other	2	2	6
Years in Five Oaks	0-5	37	32	37
	6-15	33	26	25
	16 +	30	42	37

by assigning a value of 4 if the respondent indicated that the condition was a serious problem, 3 for a moderate problem, 2 for a slight problem, and 1 for not a problem. Residents were also asked to rate Five Oaks as a very safe place (value = 4), a safe place (3), an unsafe place (2), or a very unsafe place (1). Table 4 shows that between 1992 and 1993, seriousness ratings for all conditions improved. Three of these differences in ratings, those for drugs, noisy neighbors, and traffic, were statistically significant. For the first nine conditions, the lower the score, the less serious a problem; for the safety measure, the higher the score, the more safe it was. The positive changes continued for seven of the conditions in the 1998 survey, with the changes in the ratings for drugs and prostitution being statistically significant. Noisy neighbors, housing conditions, and juvenile vandalism were all reported as more serious problems in 1998 than they were in the 1993 survey.

Another measure of residents' perceptions of crime came from a question that asked respondents to identify what they thought were the worst aspects of living in Five Oaks. Crime was mentioned by 44% of the residents in 1992, by 35% in 1993 and 38% in 1998. Both the police crime data and the residents' perceptions of crime show that the positive

TABLE 4. Perceived Seriousness of Various Problems and Safety

	Means		
	1992	1993	1998
House Thefts	2.20	2.05	2.02
Drugs	2.66[A]	2.36[B]	2.12[C]
Violence	1.86	1.73	1.66*
Other Property Crime	1.98	1.91	1.90
Juvenile Vandalism	2.17	2.09	2.12
Prostitution	2.03[A]	1.93[A]	1.45[B]
Noisy Neighbors	1.95[A]	1.69[B]	1.80[A]
Traffic	2.89[A]	1.86[B]	1.70[B]
House Maintenance	1.95	1.93	2.02
Safety	2.74	2.81	2.92

Means with different superscripts are significantly different from other years using one-way ANOVA and post hoc comparisons. If there are no superscripts in a row, then mean differences across years are nonsignficant.

effects that occurred immediately after the plan's implementation have been maintained.

While the stabilization plan was initiated in large part due to increases in crime, the goals of the plan went beyond crime reduction to include broader quality of life dimensions. Residents were asked whether the street closing plan had made the neighborhood a much better place to live, slightly better, no difference, slightly worse or much worse. While 67% of the respondents in 1993 reported that the plan had made the neighborhood a much better place (39%) or slightly better place (28%) to live, 76% in 1998 reported such improvements (50% said much better, 26% slightly better).

The plan was also designed to strengthen the residents' sense of community. Previous research on Five Oaks during the 1980s demonstrated that it was already a fairly cohesive neighborhood (Donnelly & Majka, 1996; Majka & Donnelly, 1988). While some researchers suggest that racial and economical homogeneity leads to greater neighborly ties (Bursik & Grasmick, 1993; Sampson & Groves, 1989), Five Oaks was a diverse community in which residents interacted and worked collectively in a number of ways. Interviewers asked residents a number of questions about their interaction with other residents and their involvement in neighborhood organizations. It was hoped that in strengthening the sense of community within Five Oaks, the plan would also increase residents' willingness to exercise informal social control. Many community crime prevention programs, including neighborhood watch and defensible space plans, stress the importance of strengthening communal forces that pressure people to conform to standard behavior. Since the physical changes would reduce outsiders' access to an area, it was hoped that neighbors would more easily recognize and interact with each other. Increased knowledge and interaction with neighbors can heighten residents' territoriality and sense of responsibility for what goes on in their surroundings. Table 5 shows the responses to questions addressing different aspects of community ties: knowledge of neighbors, types of interactions, organizational involvement, and commitment to the neighborhood, and residents' responsibility and care for the neighborhood.

While the plan led to an immediate reduction in crime, we realized that it might take a longer period of time to alter residents' interaction. The 1998 survey was designed to see whether there were changes in types of neighborhood interaction and commitment over a six-year period. These results can be seen in Table 5. There was no significant

TABLE 5. Indices of Community (in percent)

	1992	1993	1998
Knowledge of Neighbors by Name			
All neighbors by name	8	9	10
Most	18	24	19
Half	23	20	21
Less than half	36	41	43
None	16	7*	8
Types of Interaction			
Casual visiting	62	66	65
Visiting by invitation	55	58	56
Outside conversation	91	92	92
Taking care of home if out of town	78	75	75
Help with tasks around the house	46	37	38
Stranger Recognition			
Very easy	21	41	38
Somewhat easy	23	26	29
Somewhat difficult	27	14	22
Very difficult	30	19*	11*
Organization Involvement			
Neighborhood association	34	33	30
Church group	39	53*	53
School group	19	20	22
Commitment			
See neighborhood as:			
Real home	67	66	62
A place to live	33	34	38
Expect to be living in Five Oaks in 3 years	58	57	59
Do not expect to be living in Five Oaks	26	27	29
Do not know	16	16	12

*Chi Square significant at .01

change between 1992 and 1993 or between 1993 and 1998 in residents' knowledge of their neighbors or in various types of interaction: casual visiting with neighbors in the past few months, visiting by invitation, conversations outside their home, or help with jobs around the house. There was also no significant change between 1993 and 1998 in membership in the neighborhood association or school-related groups. Since the plan was designed to stabilize the area, we also asked two questions about residents' commitment to Five Oaks. The first asked respondents whether they felt their neighborhood was "a real home, a place where they have roots" or "just a place to live." There was no significant change in residents' responses. In each of the three years about two-thirds of the respondents said that they viewed the neighborhood as a real home. The second question measuring commitment to the neighborhood asked respondents whether they intended to be living in the neighborhood in three years. Again, there was no significant change. In each of the three years, just under 60% of the respondents expected to be living in the neighborhood in three years.

These various measures of neighborly relations, neighborhood involvement, and commitment to the neighborhood did not change significantly in the years after the plan's implementation. It is possible that such efforts simply do not bring about increased neighborliness and commitment. But other explanations, beyond the scope of this paper, are also plausible. One possible explanation is that when the NA began the process, the neighborhood already possessed a fairly high degree of cohesion and neighborliness. Neighborhoods, particularly racially and economically diverse neighborhoods, may have a peak level of cohesion which Five Oaks already possessed before the process was initiated. A second factor recognizes that all neighborhoods are dynamic entities. They are constantly changing as people move in and out, and as the neighborhood and its residents are influenced by non-neighborhood factors such as economic and family changes. Certainly, between 1992 and 1997, the neighborhood did change in various ways that might offset longer term effects that the plan might have had on neighborly interaction and residents' commitment.

The exercise of informal social control requires residents to be more watchful and involved in the neighborhood. Residents' interest and concern for the neighborhood can also be measured by their territorial behavior. Three questions addressed whether neighbors had a heightened sense of territoriality or responsibility for the neighborhood: how easy it was to recognize people who went down their street as either a resident or stranger; whether they asked a neighbor to watch their house if they went out of town; and, how they responded when they witnessed suspicious activities in the neighborhood. There was a significant change in respondents' ability to distinguish between residents and strangers on their block with most of the change occurring between 1992 and 1993. In 1992, 44% of the respondents said it was either very easy or somewhat easy to recognize someone walking or driving down their street as either a neighbor or a stranger. The street-closing plan meant that there was little cut-through traffic on most streets. After the streets were closed, most neighborhood streets were used primarily by residents. In 1993 and 1998, 67% of the residents reported that it was very easy or somewhat easy to identify someone as a neighbor or a stranger.

There was no significant change in the percent of residents who had a neighbor watch their home when they went out of town. About 75% of the respondents did this in each of the three years. There was a significant change in residents' response to suspicious activity. In 1992 and 1993, 24% and 27% of the respondents did nothing when they saw suspicious activity in the neighborhood while 46% and 41% called the police. In 1998, only 18% did nothing and 54% called the police.

CONCLUSION

This study examines the efforts of a citizen-initiated and led program to enhance the quality of life in an inner city neighborhood of Dayton, Ohio. It was designed to address some immediate problems in the neighborhood and to build a stronger sense of community for the long run. The development and implementation of the plan was spearheaded by a group of 25 to 30 leaders who worked extensively with city officials and urban planners, and involved over 500 residents in varying degrees. Some worked on subgroups or served as neighborhood captains; some only attended a few meetings. The all-volunteer NA mobilized neighborhood residents to work collectively on a plan to stabilize the neighborhood.

Rabrenovic (1996) suggested that successful NA efforts occur when neighborhood groups effectively mobilize their residents and when local governments allow significant participation in decision-making. Clearly, both of these occurred in Five Oaks. The plan brought many positive benefits to the neighborhood and its residents, including decreasing numbers of crimes. Five Oaks crime went down significantly more in the first year after the plan was implemented than it did in neighborhoods surrounding Five Oaks and in the City of Dayton as a whole. Other aspects of the quality of life, including traffic and noise, were also enhanced.

Rabrenovic (1996) also suggested that NAs were less successful in racially and economically diverse neighborhoods due to the struggles to agree on a common set of goals and strategies. It does not appear that the Five Oaks plan, or the process of developing the plan, had a significant impact on residents' sense of community, neighborly interaction, or commitment to the neighborhood. This may indicate the plan's inability to achieve one of its basic goals but may also be explained by other factors, including Five Oaks' preexisting high level of cohesion or broader factors beyond neighborhood control. These findings suggest that while crime reduction is one important component and effect of neighborhood stabilization plans, crime reduction alone is not enough to stabilize neighborhoods. Even though residents' perceived less crime in Five Oaks, there was no increase in their commitment to the neighborhood.

REFERENCES

Bellah, R., Madsen, R. Sullivan, W. M. Swidler, A. & Tipton, S. M. (1985). *Habits of the Heart: Individualism and Commitment in American Life.* Berkeley: University of California.

Berry, J., Portnoy, K. E. & Thompson, K. (1993). *The Rebirth of Urban Democracy.* Washington, D.C.: The Brookings Institution.

Bureau of Justice Statistics. (2003). *Reporting Crime to the Police, 1992-2000.* Washington, DC: U.S. Department of Justice, Office of Justice Program.

Bursik, R. J. & Grasmick, H. (1993). *Neighborhoods and Crime: The Dimensions of Effective Neighborhood Control.* New York: Lexington Books.

de Tocqueville, Alexis. (1969). *Democracy in America,* trans by G. Lawrence, Ed. By J.P. Mayer. Garden City: Anchor Books.

Donnelly, P. G. & Kimble, C. E. (1997). Community organizing, environmental change, and neighborhood crime. *Crime and Delinquency, 43,* 493-511.

Donnelly, P.G & Majka, T. J. (1998). Residents' efforts at neighborhood stabilization: Facing the challenges of inner city neighborhoods. *Sociological Forum, 13,* 189-213.

Donnelly, P. G. & Majka, T. J. (1996). Change, cohesion, and commitment in a diverse urban neighborhood. *Journal of Urban Affairs, 18,* 269-284.

Eberly, D. E. (2000). The meaning, origins, and applications of civil society. In D. E. Eberly (Ed.), *The Essential Civil Society Reader* (pp. 3-29). Lanham: Rowman and Littlefield.

Five Oaks Neighborhood Improvement Association (1993). Nomination Form, Neighborhoods USA.

Five Oaks Neighborhood Improvement Association and City of Dayton (1993). Five Oaks Neighborhood Strategic Plan.

Gurwitt, R. (Dec., 1992). A government that runs on citizen power. *Governing,* 48-54.

Helwig, R. (Feb. 25, 1993). Personal communication.

Logan, J. R. & Rabrenovic, G. (1990). Neighborhood associations: Their issues, their allies, and their opponents. *Urban Affairs Quarterly, 26,* 68-94.

Majka, T. J. & Donnelly, P. G. (1988). Cohesiveness within a heterogenous urban neighborhood: Implications for community in a diverse setting. *Journal of Urban Affairs, 10,* 141-159.

Newman, O. (1972). *Defensible space: Architectural design for crime prevention.* New York: Macmillan.

Newman, O. (1995). Defensible space: A new physical planning tool for urban revitalization. *Journal of the American Planning Association, 61,* 149-155.

Putnam, R. (January, 1995). Bowling alone: America's declining social capital. *Journal of Democracy*, 6, 65-78.

Rabrenovic, G. (1996). *Community builders: A tale of neighborhood mobilization in two cities.* Philadelphia: Temple University Press.

Sampson, R.J. & Groves, W. B. (1989). Community structure and crime: Testing social disorganization theory. *American Journal of Sociology*, *94*, 774-802.

Wuthnow, R. (2002). *Loose connections: Joining together in America's fragmented communities.* Cambridge: Harvard University Press.

Literacy for the Community, by the Community

Peter W. Dowrick
JoAnn W. L. Yuen

University of Hawai'i

SUMMARY. Literacy is a significant challenge in the U.S. and its territories, especially in low income communities where use of English language is non-standard. We developed the Actual Community Empowerment (ACE) Reading program for students at risk in such communities. ACE is a small-group tutoring program to support fluency, word recognition and decoding, and comprehension at the best pace of learning for individual, struggling readers. It has several variations (e.g., for different ages, different uses of technology), depending on local needs and re-

Address correspondence to: Peter W. Dowrick, or JoAnn W. L. Yuen, Center on Disability Studies, University of Hawai'i at Manoa, 1776 University Avenue UA4-6, Manoa, HI 96822, USA.

The authors would like to thank all the participants: community partners, students, school principals, teachers, and research assistants. They give particular acknowledgment to colleagues who took leadership roles in some of the ACE Reading studies referred to: Thomas Power, Soon Kim- Rupnow, Caryl Hitchcock, and Elisapeta Alaimaleata.

Preparation of this article was partially supported by grants from U.S. Department of Education, Office of Special Education Programs and Office of Vocational and Adult Education, although no endorsement is implied.

Some of the concepts and findings have been presented at national conferences including the 9th Biennial Conference of the Society for Community Research and Action, Las Vegas, NM, June 2003.

[Haworth co-indexing entry note]: "Literacy for the Community, by the Community." Dowrick, Peter W. and JoAnn W. L. Yuen. Co-published simultaneously in *Journal of Prevention & Intervention in the Community* (The Haworth Press, Inc.) Vol. 32, No. 1/2, 2006, pp. 81-96; and: *Community Action Research: Benefits to Community Members and Service Providers* (ed: Roger N. Reeb) The Haworth Press, Inc., 2006, pp. 81-96. Single or multiple copies of this article are available for a fee from The Haworth Document Delivery Service [1-800-HAWORTH. 9:00 a.m. - 5:00 p.m. (EST). E-mail address: docdelivery@haworthpress.com].

sources. The program has been successfully implemented in 40 locations from Philadelphia to Pohnpei, with a 95% success rate for significant reading improvement. ACE tutors are community paraprofessionals or school students with backgrounds similar to the children who receive tutoring. In the first major section of this paper, the ACE Reading Program is described and empirical research demonstrating the benefits of the program for students' literacy is reviewed. The second major section presents preliminary qualitative research evidence that paraprofessional tutors progress through recognizable stages toward increased professionalism. Recommendations for future research are provided. *[Article copies available for a fee from The Haworth Document Delivery Service: 1-800-HAWORTH. E-mail address: <docdelivery@haworthpress.com> Website: <http://www.HaworthPress.com> © 2006 by The Haworth Press, Inc. All rights reserved.]*

KEYWORDS. Actual Community Empowerment (ACE) Reading Program, literacy, tutors

Literacy remains a challenge in the United States, especially in disadvantaged communities, despite the development of many large scale literacy programs. For the most part, these programs are intended to be classroom-wide in the beginning grades. When they attend to cultural, linguistic, and economic differences, they tend to be planned and implemented in a traditional top-down educational psychology model (see Au, 2000). Such an approach requires (1) a single culture of learning to be accommodated, and (2) extensive information on that culture's learning differences. By contrast, we worked in ethnically diverse, frequently multiethnic communities, and expected to be guided toward best practices by the strengths and needs of resident cultures. That is, we used a *community response model* (Dowrick et al., 2001). Common problems across these communities were low academic achievement and unemployment.

CONTEXT OF ACE READING

Despite years of politically backed initiatives, large areas of U.S. society still struggle to achieve adequate levels of literacy. While the top tier of 15 year-olds do well by international standards (ranked 7th), the bottom 18% have very basic reading skills or less, placing the U.S. 15th overall of 31 industrialized nations and at the bottom for spread of reading scores (National Center for Education Statistics, 2001). It is commonly found in struggling schools that about 80% of the children qualify for federally subsidized lunch on the basis of family income and some 80% speak non-standard English, often as a second language. Many live in crowded homes among adults with little formal education (U.S. Census, 2000).

Approaches to literacy deficits have often been schoolwide, at least in the beginning grades. Programs such as Direct Instruction (Kame'enui, Simmons, Chard, & Dickson, 1997) and Success for All (Slavin, Madden, Dolan, & Wasik, 1996) document good outcomes when they are embraced at high cost and effort, and sometimes at the displacement of other educational priorities. Another approach is to provide supplemental support by specialists for readers who struggle the most (e.g., Clay, 1993). In communities where there are economic or linguistic minorities, there has sometimes been a cultural approach. Such programs proceed from an assumption of a unitary culture (e.g., Puerto Rican Latino, regional African-American) and educational practices are thus modified to make them "culture-friendly." For example, a promising approach initiated in India, using "cultural reciprocity," begins by recognizing the strengths of prevalent indigenous practices upon which to build western-backed educational programs (Kalyanpur, 1996).

We do not wish to denigrate the powerful good achieved by some of these approaches. But in many communities they do not provide affordable, effective, and sustainable solutions (Connell, Kubisch, Schorr, & Weiss, 1995). Overall, we find previous approaches to be too expensive and inflexible, driven by the top-down educational habits of the dominant cultures. The issue of multicultural settings has been all but ignored. In the 2000 Census, 21% of people in Hawaii identified with multiple ethnicities (vs. 2% nationally). In fact, the majority in Hawaii have significant multiple ethnicities, since more than 50% of marriages are interracial.

In summary, literacy has remained mediocre despite widespread efforts in the U.S., and most approaches may be inappropriate for those sections of society that need the greatest support. This paper presents the empirical outcomes of the Actual Community Empowerment (ACE) Reading program, which we designed to explore the effectiveness of more participatory, community-driven solutions.

Brief Description of the ACE Reading Programs

From 1998 to 2002, after its Philadelphia beginnings, we introduced the ACE Reading program in Hawaii, Pohnpei (Micronesia), Kentucky, and American Samoa. Versions of the program were also adopted in other places, including Tennessee and Oregon. These settings are highly diverse–culturally, linguistically, and economically. Some have very different educational systems. For example, Pohnpei and Samoa both have their own native languages, but use mostly English-language textbooks and teach reading in two languages in the early grades of elementary school. One site in urban Philadelphia and one in rural Kentucky had a majority of white children, but neither could be characterized as "mainstream America." Few of our participating schools in Hawaii had a single ethnic majority; most common minorities were Filipino, Native Hawaiian, and Samoan. In our U.S. schools, up to 40% of students had English as a second language (100% in other Pacific Islands) and up to 80% spoke (and wrote) nonstandard English. What most of our communities had in common included low family incomes, minimal education, many large families, and more access to television than books.

For example, Moloka'i is a small Hawaiian island, population 6,000, where three of its four elementary schools have ACE. It is rich in diversity and has deeply rooted traditions. People of Hawaiian descent are the majority (57%; Census, 2000), with smaller proportions of Filipinos, Caucasians, East Asians, and other Pacific Island peoples. Nearly 85% of students receive free or reduced-cost lunch; 16%-25% are in special education (Hawaii Department of Education, 2004). Per capita income is approximately $9,960 and 19% of the households receive Public Assistance. Almost one quarter of adults have not finished high school, and 10% have less than 9th grade education (U.S. Census, 2000). Many residents on Moloka'i, as in other Hawaiian communities, speak "Pidgin" or Hawaiian-Creole, a local dialect. It is critical for a community to have a literacy program that recognizes and values the primary language(s) while providing instruction in standard English.

The following six-element model, which is fully described by Dowrick et al. (2001; also see ACE Reading website), contains the generic, potentially universal steps that enabled us to develop ACE as the most economic and situationally respectful program possible.

1. *Identification of Needs and Strengths of the Community by the Community.* We observed and listened on site as community

members told us about issues they wanted to change, and about their struggles as well as resources.

2. *Establishing a Place in the System–by Informed Invitation.* We always introduced ACE Reading at the community's invitation, sometimes preceded by our reputation or other informational sources (e.g., news reports of ACE).

3. *Working Relationship–A Resource to the Community.* Team members were proactively responsive to the local culture, and they clearly signaled their role as one of providing empowerment rather than imposing outside expertise (e.g., training local individuals, not offering direct services).

4. *Capacity Building with Community Partners–Beyond Empowerment.* We supported local values and language in the recruitment of community members for training. If much of a community population is out of work and undereducated, these attributes may be discounted as liabilities, whereas they can be a resource. For example, we found potential tutors more available and motivated than in other communities. Some ACE 'community partners' had deficits in their own English literacy; some needed training or volunteer hours to maintain their welfare eligibility. Those who had previously been volunteers at the school described prior feelings of inadequacy and being unsure of what to do. Therefore, we developed explicit procedural protocols for community partners to become effective in specific, time-limited roles in student support (Dowrick et al., 2001; Power, Dowrick, Ginsburg-Block, & Manz, 2004).

5. *Creating Images of Future Success.* Humans learn from observing success–including one's own success and images of success not yet achieved (Dowrick, 1999). The means include: goal setting, feedforward, fostering empowerment, increasing current opportunities for success, and positive relabeling. A particular emphasis of this community response program is the principle of *feedforward*, the notion that human behavior is guided by self-images of future success. Such images may be cognitive, or constructed through stories, pictures, or computers (Dowrick, 1983, 1999). There are two related theories that support feedforward and ACE. First, Vygotsky (1978) has proposed that learning is most efficient in the *zone of proximal development* (ZPD). Information and skills are thought to be in this zone if the learner can master them with support from a coach or a slightly more able peer. Second, the initiative is based on Bandura's (1986) social-cognitive theory, spe-

cifically perceived self-efficacy, which refers to a person's belief that he or she can perform an identified task. A powerful way for individuals to acquire self-efficacy is through the observation of their own success (Dowrick, 1999; Bandura, 1997).

6. *Data-Based Evaluations, Participatory Action.* Monitoring integrity and performance keeps the project and its interventions on track and enables ongoing improvements. We used written protocols, intervention checklists, observations, regular meetings, and other frequent listening interactions to improve the program for local conditions and to give greater ownership to the constituents. Thus ACE evolved into a 10 week program, with up to four 30 minute sessions of engaging practice in oral reading and other elements most applicable to the reading level, and progress reviews every 2 weeks. Case studies have shown that paraprofessionals can deliver ACE tutoring effectively (Power et al., 2004).

Benefits to Community Children: Selective Review of Research

A number of controlled studies have been published on the outcomes of ACE Reading (e.g., Dowrick, Kim-Rupnow, & Power, 2004; Hitchcock, Prater, & Dowrick, 2004; Kim-Rupnow & Dowrick, 2001; Yuen, Dowrick, & Alaimaleata, 2004). This section provides a brief overview of the positive benefits for participating children.

We and our colleagues have completed 12 major studies on the use of ACE Reading in its various forms. Each of these studies employed either (a) an experimental design (ACE Reading group vs. a comparison group) or (b) multiple baseline designs. The main dependent variable of interest was change in oral fluency, measured with the principles of curriculum-based assessment (Fuchs, Fuchs, Hosp, & Jenkins, 2001), which revealed differences of educational and statistical significance in all studies. Typically, we targeted the 15% to 20% of readers who were struggling the most in a grade level, with the goal of improving their reading levels, so that they could succeed in class. Ninety-five percent of students met this goal in one semester or one year. There were also significant improvements in vocabulary, comprehension, decoding skills, classroom behavior, and attitudes toward reading (i.e., perseverance).

In a number of instances, students were no longer classified as "special education" or "at risk" following participation in ACE for one year (Dowrick et al., 2004; Hitchcock et al., 2004). In implementation projects, where we provided materials and limited consultation for teachers to run ACE with community support, similar results were obtained. For example, in a summer program with 18 elementary school students, reading improvements were evident in 3 weeks, with 10 of them improving one to two grade levels. In a 6-month afterschool program using tutors from the local high school, 12 first graders improved in reading by almost a grade level, and 12 older elementary school children improved by almost two grade levels, even though these students were selected because they had the slowest progress in literacy in their school.

Two versions have emerged as particularly viable for the lower elementary grades: ACE Reading with books and paper products only and Computer ACE (using multimedia). The latter proves most popular where computer access is novel, and because students as young as those in fifth grade can be successful tutors. Consequently, the state of Pohnpei in Micronesia has adopted ACE as one of its main afterschool programs. The initial pilots produced very favorable results; for instance, after 6 months of tutoring, the reading scores of three students improved from the bottom of the third grade level to the top of the third grade level. The first Computer ACE study analyzed in urban Honolulu indicated improvements in oral fluency three times as great as the level of improvement obtained by students receiving regular classroom reading instructions over the same time period (Kim-Rupnow & Dowrick, 2001).

On an outer island in Hawaii, in a study of ACE Reading incorporating video feedforward, other benefits were noted. The primary investigator interviewed teachers, parents, and tutors after the intervention (Hitchcock et al., 2004). She found that the gains in reading generalized across environments (afterschool, classroom, home), and were associated with improved behavior and emotional responses to normal stresses of the classroom and family life at home.

Where ACE has been active for multiple years, with an emphasis on kindergarten through second grade, changes in third grade reading scores on the Stanford Achievement Test (SAT) have been significant. In our first school in Hawaii, the percentage of students in the so-called average and above categories increased from 27% to 74% (1997-2000); another school, with less room to improve, increased from 63% to 76% in a recent implementation of ACE (2000-2003). In a comparable neighboring school, third grade SAT scores declined (70% to 66%) from 2002 to 2003 (Hawaii Department of Education, 2004).

BENEFITS OF ACE READING PROGRAM
FOR COMMUNITY TUTORS:
PRELIMINARY QUALITATIVE FINDINGS

This section presents preliminary findings from qualitative studies suggesting that paraprofessional tutors in the ACE Reading Program progress through recognizable stages toward increased levels of professionalism.

Method

Given the favorable results of ACE Reading programs, we undertook qualitative studies to better understand the implementation process on site, the program's connections to the local community, and the program's significance to other communities (Borg & Gall, 1989). We used three methods of research: participant observation, content analysis, and personal interview. In an attempt to collect reliable data and triangulate the results (LeCompte & Goetz, 1982), these qualitative studies were conducted over a 4-year period in five different communities, with different age groups, and at different times over a 4-year period.

Samples and Procedures

Elementary School Tutors. Tutors consisted of 10 sixth graders (5 males and 5 females) between 11 and 12 years of age (median age = 11.6), and race/ethnicity included 5 Filipino, 4 Hawaiian, and 1 Micronesian. Teachers selected sixth grade students using the following criteria: up-to-date with academic work; reading at grade level; participating in extracurricular activities (e.g., band, teacher assistant); and considered "trustworthy" and "responsible" by their teacher. Students could be removed from tutoring assignments if they were "benched" (placed on detention or faced disciplinary action), needed to concentrate on academics and homework, or because of excessive competing extracurricular activities.

The second author trained and mentored students to become tutors for first graders. Data was collected through observations and training interactions during the course of tutoring and debriefing from April 2003 through May 2003, a relatively short intervention. We provided 2 hours of Computer ACE (C'ACE) Reading tutor training, 2 hours of software/computer time with tutees, and on-the-job mentoring. Data were kept in the form of a daily journal.

High School Tutors. Tutors included 8 high school students (3 males and 5 females) between the ages of 15 and 17 (median age = 16.1). Regarding race/ethnicity, 5 were Caucasian and 3 were African American. At the Kentucky elementary school, the local ACE staff recruited and trained tutors from the neighboring high school, enabling students to fulfill their service-learning requirements (Barr, 2002). Teachers identified the six most struggling readers in each of four classes and arranged for them to receive tutoring from the high school students. Tutor data were collected using open-ended questions regarding tutors' perceived benefits of the tutoring for both students and tutors.

Adult Community Tutors. Interviews were conducted with 2 female Micronesian tutors (35 and 45 years of age) in Pohnpei, 2 female (1 Samoan and 1 Hawaiian) tutors (45 and 55 years of age) in Kalihi, and 3 female Samoan tutors in American Samoa (45, 47, and 50 years of age). The same individual (first language Samoan, second language English) conducted these seven interviews and transcribed the data. All interviews were in English, except those collected in American Samoa. The following is a sample interview question: "What did you hope to gain from being a tutor?" For a detailed description, see Yuen et al. (2004).

Analysis of Preliminary Qualitative Data

Given the diverse locations, populations, and ages of tutors, there was an attempt to identify the similarities and differences in tutors' perceptions of their work experiences. Data were analyzed and drafted into narrative form by the second author, using a six-step protocol:

1. Examine content of interviews, observations, and surveys in order to identify similarities among tutor's perceptions of their work experiences;
2. Examine underlined key words and phrases, and create rough descriptors;
3. Refine and combine categories, by sample, including key quotations;
4. Confirm perceptions, concepts, and understanding with the source (i.e., interviewer, transcriber, trainer, or teacher);
5. Develop categories within each site;
6. Combine categories across sites to find common elements.

Results

The above qualitative analysis revealed five experiential categories that were distinct from one another in two important ways: (1) in the degree of tutor responsibility (to another person, self, and community) and (2) in the level of interaction between the tutor and the learning environment/student. In step 6, we concluded it was possible to identify five distinct categories that may reflect the development in the tutor's progress toward professionalism. At each categorical level, the tutor was successful and the ACE system benefited the student's literacy development. At higher levels, however, the tutor appeared to contribute more and to gain additional professional experience. The five categories identified in this preliminary qualitative analysis, which were common to all ACE sites, suggested that ACE tutors may progress through a number of recognizable stages towards increasingly higher level of professionalism.

Process-Dedicated Tutors. Process-dedicated tutors waited for instructions and asked for assistance with each new, unfamiliar step. Tutors showed less initiative and required continual support and encouragement from mentors. For example, one tutor received a computer message that asked him if he wanted to reset the computer to lower resolution for the software he was loading. Another tutor advised him to "hit yes," but he did not proceed until a mentor intervened. In general, comments and questions continued to reflect procedural issues (e.g., "Do I start now?"), and were not limited to the first days of training.

Process-dedicated tutors tended toward one-way interaction with students and asked to work with only one tutee (the ACE protocol is designed for at least two tutees). The tutor taught and the tutee followed.

Self-Focused Tutors. The first two categories were centered on the tutor and tutoring procedures. For example, a tutor described his role as follows, "I sounded out words they needed help on, we went over everything that was asked. We read the book three times. We played all the games to help them learn more." This is where similarities between the first two categories ended. Self-focused tutors were problem solvers, they liked to work with minimal supervision, and they modified protocols and procedures to suit personal needs (e.g., play with the computer, take a break from classes or from "routines" and "household chores").

Self-focused tutors tried to control the interactions (i.e., the pace of the tutoring, with whom they tutored, and so on). Two tutors competed to determine which tutee was reading faster. Even so, the tutor acted as if he or she was not responsible for the tutee's outcomes, and became bored if a student was not advancing or needed to repeat reading material. Another tutor wanted to advance his tutee from one to two books a day, even though the tutee was not able to keep up. He said, "My kid is too hard, I want an easier one, one that reads better."

Student-Centered Tutors. Student-centered tutors put the well-being and outcomes of their tutees first. They were engaged with students and ACE protocols. They felt responsible for the outcomes and attempted to control the learning environment. One tutor buffered a chaotic classroom environment by huddling with her tutee. With an arm around the back of chair, she used her body to block out classroom noise. Within the C'ACE structure, student-centered tutors identified ways to improve teaching, and they attempted to adjust the program to the tutee's needs and abilities. One tutor suggested, "If the children working in the program are faster than others, it [the software] should be sped up a little." With encouragement and training, tutors were able to assess the potential of tutees, "I feel [tutee's name] can read better [than he does]."

Student-centered tutors were able to tutor two students at a time and felt responsible for the process of learning and the accomplishments. One student noted benefiting from being a tutor because, "The little kids were my responsibility and it made me feel good helping them to get to their reading level." Two tutors felt they could have been more successful, given more time. One tutor commented, "If I had more time it would have been better . . . I could only work with them for about 30-35 minutes." He believed more learning could have occurred with longer tutoring sessions. Another tutor stated, "If I had started working with [tutee] earlier, [she] would have been at a higher book."

Generalizing Tutors. Generalizing tutors formed partnerships with their tutees, took responsibility, showed initiative, creatively solved problems, and generalized experiences to other settings. For example, one tutor described how adult tutors created a process that was shared by tutor and tutee. She believed the C'ACE protocols were easy for any parent to follow, "Filipino parent or any type of nationality you train them how to follow the protocol they won't miss a thing. It's really easy. It doesn't need education to really know how to do that. The protocol is in my brain. I follow the protocol exactly . . ." and tutees "would stop the tutors and remind the tutors, 'Hey we missed a step'."

Generalizing tutors embraced responsibility ("Teach me that [probing] next!") and involvement in ACE (e.g., tutoring, probing, handing out rewards), apparently wanting to learn. One tutor commented, "I learn from the school, the teachers. So working together within the school system is good and I recommend it for a lot of parents and the end of the day they'll reward themselves." Some tutors wanted to tutor more students and manipulate the environment to meet the goals of C'ACE. One tutor asked, "Why can't we tutor in the computer center, there's lots [more] room. . . ." Another tutor supported this idea, " . . . there is room on the floor for students who don't behave."

They appeared more outcome-driven and manipulated the protocol at the request of a tutee. One tutor asked to work longer with a tutee who had difficulty concentrating and was identified as "special ed." The tutee wanted more time to memorize words that he had found to be confusing ("Mit," "Mat," and "Raft"), so the tutor spent additional time reviewing the material with the tutee, and then provided more time for the tutee to practice alone. That afternoon the tutee was heard repeating the words: "Raft, Raft, Raft; Mat, Mat, Mat; Mit, Mit, Mit." The same tutor spoke to the older siblings of another tutee to get insight into how to manage him in the classroom. She felt that she was "the best one to tutor him" because she understood his "angry behavior" and believed she could control him because "I know his sister and he will listen to me."

The generalizing tutor identified elements of the task, offered information, ideas and insights, and adjusted tutoring to meet the tutee's needs. Adult tutors in Kalihi were concerned about comprehension. They were unsure if their students did not know words or if they did not understand English so they taught ACE using Samoan words. A Kalihi tutor said,

> Oh yeah, I had quite a few Samoan students, those who didn't know their ABC fully. . . . I didn't know whether they understand English or not. So what I did, I used both English and Samoan to see what part they understand better. . . kids growing up here, they understand English more than Samoan. I was able to teach them in the English language too.

Community-Directed Tutors. In this category, we observed an extension of the generalization process. Such tutors seemed to become aware of their participation in a bigger picture, and appeared to be positively changed by it. They made systematic generalizations from ACE to other settings and to their own lives. Community-directed tutors were self-reflective. Prior to ACE, these tutors described their child-parent interactions as "I would hardly read books to my son" or "I would watch them read." ACE promoted interdependence between children and parents around educational activities. Tutors no longer assumed passive roles toward the education of their own children; instead, they were more active, interactive and supportive. One tutor stated:

> I really learn a lot after volunteering in education, because I thought school–never mind, I don't care. But when I joined ACE, I see that it was really important to teach my child for education. She has to learn. I know it was very hard . . . it will take time to make it easy for them. But my child, she didn't want to go back to school anymore. She was sick [has special needs]. I told her, you have to go back to school. You don't have to quit, you have to move on, so that you can move on to the next level to help you because one day if I die, you can take care of yourself. I cannot take care of her all the time. . . .

After observing the benefits of ACE, one tutor envisioned success not yet achieved in the migration of people from Samoa to Hawaii:

> I think it will be very effective, because of the fact that most of the Samoan kids that come over here (Hawaii), they understand English. So I think if we bring in a program to the Samoan people for the Samoan students, it will work. Because if they move from Samoa to Hawaii, they would already know how to speak English already. From there they can go, follow the curriculum. Right now, children from Samoa only speak Samoan, they don't know how to speak English. But if we bring home some kind of program where they can learn from K [kindergarten] all the way into fifth grade or more, or even the teen years, I think it'll be very effective.

Another tutor generalized her tutoring experiences to similar situations, "I can [now] teach my little siblings how to break down words as they read, and develop games for them."

Community-directed tutors also became advocates of ACE and literacy. Not only did they want to tutor more children, they also wanted to recruit and train community partners. One tutor recommended "training parents be become reading tutors," and this tutor indicated that, "I've asked parents to come and sit in. I encourage them to use the routine at home because it has a structure that you can use with all your children at home."

GENERAL DISCUSSION AND CONCLUSION

We developed–that is, we fostered the evolution of–the ACE Reading program across a range of communities, with positive outcomes for participants who received or delivered services. The program, and even the target of "literacy," was developed in response to community requests, not selected and provided by outside experts. We incorporated scientific expertise, but only as it could be adopted and adapted to fit available resources. ACE managers selected and supported tutors based on three criteria (i.e., read at a fourth grade level, work well with children, and reliable). Community-based tutors represented an available, affordable resource. Tutors served as mentors and role models for children, with whom they shared common backgrounds.

This paper reviewed evidence that the ACE Reading Program has positive effects on students' literacy. In addition, we identified five categories of tutors, or levels of professionalism, in the ACE program, and these categories differed regarding (1) the extent to which tutors accepted responsibility for outcomes, and (2) the nature of interaction between the tutor and the student (or learning environment). These five tutor categories were labeled: process-dedicated tutors; self-focused tutors; student-centered tutors; generalizing tutors; and community-directed tutors. These preliminary results of qualitative research suggest that paraprofessional tutors may progress through recognizable stages toward increased professionalism.

The following are some recommendations for future research focused on identifying the benefits of the ACE Reading Program for paraprofessional tutors. First, in order to confirm the five categories of tutors noted above, replication studies are needed. Second, if the tutor categories are confirmed, then research is needed to determine the utility of these categories for the assessment and training of community tutors. Third, prospective longitudinal research is needed to determine the extent to which the identified categories are developmental in nature. Fourth, another topic for prospective longitudinal research is to examine the extent to which literacy is enhanced by teaching it. That is, what is the potential for tutors, whether of school-age or adult, to benefit in their own literacy skills as they help others? Finally, prospective longitudinal research would help us to better understand other potential benefits to ACE tutors. For instance, unemployed adults who become ACE tutors are earning extra money, enhancing their resumes (and sometimes obtaining employment), improving the education of their own families, and gaining respect in the community.

In conclusion, Adrienne Rich (1986) spoke about the inequities of culture, "When someone with the authority of a teacher, say, describes the world and you are not in it, there is a moment of psychic disequilibrium, as if you looked into a mirror and saw nothing" (p. 198). We want to create positive images of future success, such that when someone of authority describes a student's world, the student is in it, and the student experiences that moment of psychic empowerment, as if he or she looked into a mirror and saw someone special (Yuen & Shaughnessy, 2000). Thus, we will continue to apply principles of community responsiveness to our intervention research, which focuses on the future development of the community, by the community.

REFERENCES

ACE Reading website. (2004). http://www.cds.hawaii.edu/reading/ accessed 29 August 2004.

Au, K.H. (2000). A multicultural perspective on policies for improving literacy achievement: Equity and excellence. In M.L. Kamil, P.B. Mosenthal, P.D. Pearson, & R. Barr (Eds.), *Handbook of reading research* (Vol. 3) (pp. 835-870). Mahwah, NJ: Erlbaum.

Bandura, A. (1986). *Social foundations of thought and action: A social cognitive theory.* Englewood Cliffs, NJ: Prentice Hall.

Bandura, A. (1997). *Self-efficacy: The exercise of control.* New York: Freeman.

Barr, J. (2002, March). Bardstown high school students are 'ACEs' in tutoring primary students struggling to read. *Kentucky Teacher, 4.*

Borg, W.K., & Gall, M.D. (1989). *Educational research: An introduction* (5th ed.). White Plains, NY: Longman.

Clay, M.M. (1993). *Reading Recovery: A guidebook for teachers in training.* Portsmouth, NH: Heinemann.

Connell, J.P., Kubisch, A.C., Schorr, L.B., & Weiss, C. (1995). *New approaches to evaluating community initiatives.* Washington, DC: Aspen Institute.

Dowrick, P.W. (1983). Self-modelling. In P.W. Dowrick & S.J. Biggs (Eds.), *Using video: Psychological and social applications* (pp. 105-124). Chichester, UK: Wiley.

Dowrick, P.W. (1999). A review of self modeling and related interventions. *Applied and Preventive Psychology, 8,* 23-39.

Dowrick, P.W., Kim-Rupnow, W.S., & Power, T.J. (2004). Video feedforward for reading. *Journal of Special Education,* accepted for publication.

Dowrick, P.W., Power, T.J., Manz, P.H., Ginsburg-Block, M., Leff, S.S., & Kim-Rupnow, S. (2001). Community responsiveness: Examples from under-resourced urban schools. *Journal of Prevention and Intervention in the Community, 21*(2), 71-90.

Fuchs, L.S., Fuchs, D., Hosp, M.K., & Jenkins, J.R. (2001). Oral reading fluency as an indicator of reading competence: A theoretical, empirical, and historical analysis. *Scientific Studies of Reading, 3,* 239-256

Hawai'i Department of Education. (2004). *School status and improvement report.* Honolulu: Author.

Hitchcock, C., Prater, M.A., & Dowrick, P.W. (2004). Reading comprehension and fluency: Examining the effects of tutoring and video self modeling on first grade students with reading difficulties. *Learning Disability Quarterly, 27,* 89-103.

Kalyanpur, M. (1996). The influences of western special education on community-based services in India. *Disability and Society, 11,* 249-269.

Kame'enui, E.J., Simmons, D.C., Chard, D., & Dickson, S. (1997). Direct-Instruction reading. In S.A. Stahl & D.A. Hayes (Eds.), *Instructional models in reading* (pp. 59-84). Hillsdale, NJ: Erlbaum.

Kim-Rupnow, W.S., & Dowrick, P.W. (2001). Computer-enhanced tutoring and self modeling for early reading acquisition. *Journal of Asia-Pacific Special Education, 1*(2), 13-18.

LeCompte, M.D., & Goetz, J.P. (1982). Problems of reliability and validity in ethnographic research. *Review of Educational Research, 521,* 31-60.

National Center for Education Statistics (NCES). (2001). *Outcomes of learning: Results from the 2000 Program for International Student Assessment of 15-year-olds in reading, mathematics, and science literacy.* Washington, DC: US Department of Education: Office of Educational Research and Improvement.

Power, T.J., Dowrick, P.W., Ginsburg-Block, M., & Manz, P.H. (2004). Partnership-based community-assisted early intervention for literacy: An application of the participatory intervention model. *Journal of Behavioral Education, 13,* 93-115.

Rich, A.C. (1986). *Blood, bread and poetry: Selected prose 1979-1985,* New York: Norton.

Slavin, R.E., Madden, N. A., Dolan, L.J., & Wasik, B.A. (1996). *Every child, every school: Success for all.* Newbury Park, CA: Corwin.

U.S. Census Bureau. (2000). *Census of population.* Washington, DC: U.S. Government Printing Office.

Vygotsky, L.S. (1978). *Mind in society.* Cambridge, MA: Harvard University Press.

Yuen, J.W.L., Dowrick, P.W., & Alaimaleata, E.T. (2004). Using a community response model in literacy education. *Research on the Education of Asian and Pacific-Americans (Vol. 3)* (in press).

Yuen, J.W.L., & Shaughnessy, B. (2001). Cultural empowerment: Tools to engage and retain postsecondary students with disabilities. *Journal of Vocational Rehabilitation, 16,* 199-207.

PART II:
COMMUNITY ACTION RESEARCH:
BENEFITS TO SERVICE PROVIDERS

The Community Service
Self-Efficacy Scale:
Further Evidence of Reliability and Validity

Roger N. Reeb

University of Dayton

SUMMARY. The Community Service Self-Efficacy Scale (CSSES) measures " . . . the individual's confidence in his or her own ability to make clinically significant contributions to the community through ser-

Address correspondence to: Roger N. Reeb, Department of Psychology, University of Dayton, Dayton, OH 45469-1430 (E-mail: roger.reeb@notes.udayton.edu).

The author wishes to thank Ronald M. Katsuyama for his helpful comments on an earlier version of this manuscript.

[Haworth co-indexing entry note]: "The Community Service Self-Efficacy Scale: Further Evidence of Reliability and Validity." Reeb, Roger N. Co-published simultaneously in *Journal of Prevention & Intervention in the Community* (The Haworth Press, Inc.) Vol. 32, No. 1/2, 2006, pp. 97-113; and: *Community Action Research: Benefits to Community Members and Service Providers* (ed: Roger N. Reeb) The Haworth Press, Inc., 2006, pp. 97-113. Single or multiple copies of this article are available for a fee from The Haworth Document Delivery Service [1-800-HAWORTH, 9:00 a.m. - 5:00 p.m. (EST). E-mail address: docdelivery@haworthpress.com].

vice" (Reeb et al., p. 48). Three studies reported in this article replicate and extend past CSSES research. With regard to reliability, results replicate past research in demonstrating internal consistency and temporal consistency. Convergent validity was demonstrated by the finding that, as hypothesized, the CSSES correlated moderately with a measure of general self-efficacy. As hypothesized, the correlation between the CSSES and a measure of social desirability was low in magnitude and non-significant, demonstrating discriminant validity. Regarding gender differences, females tended to score somewhat higher than males on the CSSES. With respect to construct validity, CSSES scores changed in the hypothesized direction in response to an intervention. While past CSSES research focused on college students, one study reported in this paper shows that the CSSES is useful in studying adolescents, including those with psychosocial adjustment problems. *[Article copies available for a fee from The Haworth Document Delivery Service: 1-800-HAWORTH. E-mail address: <docdelivery@haworthpress.com> Website: <http://www.HaworthPress.com> © 2006 by The Haworth Press, Inc. All rights reserved.]*

KEYWORDS. Community Service Self-Efficacy Scale, service-learning, program evaluation, self-efficacy, community service

The Community Service Self-Efficacy Scale (CSSES) was developed and validated by Reeb, Katsuyama, Sammon, and Yoder (1998) to be used in research and program evaluation in the area of service-learning. The CSSES, which is presented in its entirety by Reeb et al. (1998), measures " . . . the individual's confidence in his or her own ability to make clinically significant contributions to the community through service" (p. 48). In a critique of psychometric instruments used in service-learning research, Bringle, Phillips, and Hudson (2004) conclude that " . . . the CSSES is significant as a scale developed for service learning with good theoretical rationale, promising psychometric characteristics, and potential utility as a moderator variable, mediating variable, and outcome variable" (pp. 101-102).

The present paper contributes to the empirical literature on this psychometric instrument. The paper is organized into four sections: In the first section, a brief overview of research and theory on the self-efficacy construct is provided, and the rationale for developing the CSSES is discussed. The second section provides a review of past research examining the psychometric properties of the CSSES. In the third section, the results of three new empirical studies examining the reliability and validity of the CSSES are presented. Finally, the fourth section summarizes empirical findings and provides general directions for future research on the CSSES.

THEORETICAL BACKGROUND AND RATIONALE

The Self-Efficacy Construct: An Overview of Research and Theory

Self-efficacy, a theoretical construct derived from Bandura's social-cognitive theory, is defined as follows: "an expectation of personal mastery . . . " (1977, p. 191); a "self-appraisal of operative capability" (1982, p. 123); "a conviction that one can successfully execute the behavior required to produce [desired] outcomes"(1977, p. 193); or " . . . a belief in one's capabilities to organize and execute the courses of action required to manage prospective situations" (1995, p. 2). As reviewed by Bandura (1997), almost three decades of research has provided support for his original hypothesis that " . . . expectations of personal efficacy determine whether coping behavior is initiated, how much effort will be expended, and how long it will be sustained in the face of obstacles and aversive experiences . . . " (1977, p. 191). In addition, across a variety of situations, circumstances, and populations, the following pattern of results is obtained in research: First, self-efficacy for coping in a given situation tends to improve as an individual receives an intervention designed to enhance coping competence. Second, while post-intervention self-efficacy is positively correlated with future performance accomplishments in the situation, it is inversely related to anxiety (and other debilitating emotions) during performance. Most studies show that, relative to an individual's actual performance attainments during an intervention, the person's self-efficacy level at post-intervention is a better predictor of subsequent performance accomplishments (Bandura, 1997), further suggesting that self-efficacy plays a major role in the initiation and persistence of coping behavior.

To conceptualize how developmental changes in self-efficacy occur, Bandura (1978) proposed the principle of reciprocal determinism, which maintains that self-efficacy, behavior, and environmental factors transact and influence one another in a bidirectional fashion. Bandura (1978, p. 346) writes: "In the . . . process of reciprocal determinism, behavior, internal personal factors, and environmental influences all operate as interlocking determinants of each other . . . in a triadic reciprocal interaction. . . . For example, people's efficacy . . . expectations influence how they behave, and the environmental effects created by their actions in turn alter their expectations. . . . " Given the principle of reciprocal determinism, the following pattern would be expected in the area of community service-learning: a student with high self-efficacy for community service would be more likely than a student with low self-efficacy to pursue service-learning opportunities; once the student with high self-efficacy becomes involved in service, he or she would exhibit high levels of effort and perseverance, even when obstacles and failures are initially encountered; in turn, the favorable service experiences and outcomes, created in part by the student's behavior, would reinforce and further improve his or her self-efficacy for community service. Conversely, if a student with low self-efficacy for community service became involved in a service-learning project, he or she would be expected to become frustrated easily and lack persistence in the face of obstacles; in turn, the negative service experiences and failures, created in part by the student's behavior, would lead to a further decline in his or her self-efficacy for community service.

Rationale for Development of the CSSES

The rationale for development of the CSSES was threefold. First, the construct of self-efficacy is inherently pertinent to the goals of service-learning. As argued by Miller (1997), "One of the explicit goals of service-learning is to help students recognize that they can use knowledge gained in service-learning experiences to make the world a better place" (p. 16).

Second, it seemed clear that service-learning research on the self-efficacy construct would fill a significant void in the literature. While most of the psychometric instruments used in service-learning research (see Bringle et al., 2004) focused on such domains as motives (e.g., reasons for engaging in community service), values (e.g., social responsibility or commitment to help others), perceived community needs (e.g., beliefs regarding the extent to which community members need help from volunteers), or attitudes toward community service (e.g., beliefs about whether people have a *duty* to serve), there had been a dearth of research examining the construct of self-efficacy (confidence or sense of competence) for community service. Bandura's (1997) distinction between self-efficacy expectations and outcome expectations is helpful in illustrating the difference between self-efficacy and other constructs of interest in service-learning research: " . . . self-efficacy is a judgment of one's ability to organize and execute given types of performances, whereas an outcome expectation is a judgment of the likely consequences such performances will produce ..." (p. 21). For instance, consider a student with a high sense of social responsibility accompanied by a belief that everyone has a duty to serve. Such an individual may also firmly believe that a certain set of actions (e.g., assisting in the implementation of a community-based diversion program for conduct-disordered youth) would address a perceived need in the community, but if the student has serious doubts regarding his or her capacity to perform the set of action, this belief may not motivate the student to pursue the service opportunity.

Third, as reviewed by Reeb et al. (1998), the few studies that did examine self-efficacy in the service-learning literature (e.g., Miller, 1997) used measures with little or no demonstrated psychometric properties and, since these measures consisted of only one or two items, reliability was questionable. Further, items on these early scales tended to be global in nature (i.e., pertaining to a general sense of power to impact the world), and so validity was also in question. As noted by Miller (1997) and Reeb et al. (1998), a low score on a global item may reflect a sense of realism as opposed to a belief that one does not have an ability to contribute to his or her immediate community through service. Thus, it became clear that advancements in our understanding of the role of self-efficacy in service-learning required development and validation of a psychometric instrument to measure the construct.

PSYCHOMETRIC PROPERTIES OF THE CSSES: OVERVIEW OF PAST PUBLISHED RESEARCH

Reeb et al. (1998) reported the results of three studies that replicated and complemented one another in demonstrating reliability and validity for the CSSES. The findings are summarized below.

Internal Consistency

For each of the three studies, coefficient alpha was over .90 for the CSSES, demonstrating internal consistency for the instrument. Across the three studies, item-total correlation coefficients ranged from .68 to .78 in Study 1, .62 to .79 in Study 2, and .88 to .95 in Study 3.

Temporal Consistency

Study 2 examined test-retest (pre- to post-semester) reliability for the CSSES with students who were not involved in service-learning during that particular semester. As expected, the coefficient of stability was high in magnitude and statistically significant ($r = .62, p = .001$), and the pre- to post-semester mean difference in CSSES scores was not statistically significant.

Factor Structure

With regard to construct validity, Study 1 conducted a factor analysis ($N = 676$) of CSSES items and items of the Social Responsibility Inventory (SRI; Markus, Howard, & King, 1993). As hypothesized, items of the CSSES loaded heavily on a separate unique factor, with item loadings ranging from .67 to .81. Thus, results suggested that the CSSES is unidimensional.

Discriminant Validity

In the factor analysis research reviewed above, CSSES items did not load on other factors, and SRI items did not load on the CSSES factor, and this pattern of findings provides some evidence of discriminant validity.

Criterion-Related (Concurrent) Validity

The method of contrasted groups was used to examine criterion-related validity. Study 1 found that students who participated in each of three types of service (i.e., extracurricular, summer, and course-related) during past year had higher CSSES scores than students who were not involved in that particular type of service. Further, a linear effect for participation was observed: students in three types of service programs during the past year had higher CSSES scores than those who participated in only two; students in two types of service programs scored higher on the CSSES relative to those who participated in only one; and students in one type of service program had higher CSSES scores compared to those involved in none. In addition, multiple regression analyses indicated that, relative to a list of other factors pertinent to service-learning, items of the CSSES accounted for the greatest variance in measures of both involvement and satisfaction in each type of past service (extracurricular, summer, and course-related).

Finally, consistent with research showing that self-efficacy influences initiation and persistence of behavior (Bandura, 1997), Study 2 found that students who pursued a course-related service-learning opportunity had significantly higher CSSES scores relative to those who did not pursue service-learning. This finding provided further evidence of criterion-related (concurrent) validity.

Sensitivity to Intervention Effects

Construct validity is established for a measure with the gradual accumulation of evidence from different sources over time, and each type of evidence presented above is pertinent to construct validity. Another source of data for construct validity is provided by studies demonstrating that scores on a measure change in the hypothesized direction in response to an intervention (Anastasi & Urbina, 1997; Cronbach & Meehl, 1955). Consistent with research indicating that self-efficacy improves over the course on an intervention, Study 2 hypothesized a pre- to post-semester increase in CSSES scores for service-learning students but not for students not participating in service-learning. However, students who pursued the service-learning opportunity had extremely high CSSES scores at pre-semester, perhaps creating a *ceiling effect* that precluded an adequate test of the hypothesis. Thus, service-learning students maintained high CSSES scores from pre- to post-semester, but their CSSES scores did not significantly increase over the course of the semester. While it seems likely that this finding is due to a *ceiling effect*, Reeb et al. (1998) concluded that "further research is needed to determine the ways in which service-learning experiences influence students' perceptions of self-efficacy in the area of community service" (p. 55). Some of the new findings presented in the next section are relevant to this matter.

In Study 3, Reeb et al. (1998) used a version of the CSSES that assesses students' retrospective perceptions of a course's contribution to their self-efficacy for community service (i.e., *"This course increased or strengthened my confidence that, in the future, I will be able to . . . "*). This CSSES version is useful in situations where (a) pre-semester testing is not possible, or (b) students already have extremely high CSSES at pre-semester (perhaps creating a *ceiling effect* that precludes an examination of change). Using this retrospective version of the CSSES, Study 3 found that students who participated in service-learning during the semester obtained higher CSSES scores compared to those who did not participate in service-learning.

COMMUNITY SERVICE SELF-EFFICACY SCALE: NEW RESEARCH FINDINGS

Study 1

In their critique of psychometric instruments for service-learning research, Bringle et al. (2004) noted that, " . . . there is no information available about the scale's correlation with social desirability or acquiescent response bias" (p. 101). However, a study presented by Reeb et al. (1999) found that the correlation between the CSSES and the Marlowe-Crowne Social Desirability Scale was low in magnitude and not statistically significant. Nevertheless, the extent to which CSSES scores reflect social desirability or an acquiescent response bias is an important issue in the process of establishing construct validity for a measure of this kind (Cronbach & Meehl, 1955), and so Study 1 attempted to replicate the finding reported by Reeb et al. (1999). In addition, Study 1 attempted to replicate research demonstrating that the CSSES has internal consistency (Reeb et al. (1998), and it also examined gender differences in CSSES scores.

Sample and Procedure. In a group testing format, a number of measures, including the CSSES and the Marlowe-Crowne Social Desirability Scale (Crowne & Marlowe, 1964), were administered to 394 undergraduate students (115 males, 279 females) between the ages of 17 and 22 years ($M = 18.62$; $SD = .80$). The CSSES is a 10-item scale, with scores ranging from 1 (*quite uncertain*) to 10 (*certain*) for each item. The Marlowe-Crowne is a 33-item (*true* or *false*) scale. The sample consisted of 360 (91.1%) European-Americans, 18 (4.5%) African-Americans, 5 (1.3%) Hispanic-Americans, 5 (1.3%) Asian-Americans, and 7 (1.8%) Other.

Results and Discussion. Consistent with past research, internal consistency for the CSSES was demonstrated (alpha coefficient = .95), and none of the items detracted from internal consistency (alpha coefficient). Item-total correlations (corrected) ranged from .71 to .83.

Regarding gender differences in CSSES scores, females ($n = 279$, $M = 7.78$, $SD = 1.63$) tended to score higher on the CSSES relative to males

(n = 115, M = 7.06. SD = 1.91), $t(392)$ = 3.78, $p < .001$. Gender differences in CSSES scores is further examined and discussed in Study 3 of the present paper.

Consistent with results presented by Reeb et al. (1999), the correlation between the CSSES and the Marlowe-Crowne Social Desirability Scale was low in magnitude ($r = .09$) and not statistically significant ($p > .05$). The correlation coefficients between specific CSSES items and the total score of the Marlowe-Crowne Social Desirability Scale were low in magnitude and ranged from .008 to .15. Thus, the notion that CSSES scores reflect social desirability seems implausible. Since the CSSES items have a high level of *face validity*, and it would seem that the attribute being measured is one that many people would find to be *desirable*, attempts to further rule out the possibility that CSSES scores reflect *impression management* or *self-deception* may be justified, and a researcher could do this by either replicating the present finding and/or examining the correlation between the CSSES and other measures of social desirability. Further, if this issue is a concern in research, then an investigator could administer a measure of social desirability along with the CSSES and statistically control for (i.e., partial out) variance associated social desirability.

Study 2

As noted earlier, evidence of construct validity for a measure is provided by studies demonstrating that scores on the measure change in the hypothesized direction in response to an intervention (Anastasi & Urbina, 1997; Cronbach & Meehl, 1955). The primary purpose of this study was to examine the hypothesis that conduct-disordered adolescents would show improvements in CSSES scores as they participated in a community-based diversion program (CBDP). This particular CBDT, as described by Pratt, Smith, Reigelsperger, O'Connor, Saum, Baker, and Reeb (2003), has some similarities to other well-established programs for troubled youth (Davidson, Redner, & Mitchell, 1990; also see reviews by Kazdin, 1995, 1997). However, one component of this particular CBDT is an emphasis on *work therapy*, in which the adolescents become involved in community service. Russo (1974, p. 531) noted that work therapy is designed to " . . . improve the self-concept of delinquents by giving them an opportunity to help others." In the paper by Pratt et al. (2003), it was argued that, since work therapy is "conceptually-related" to service-learning, research demonstrating the beneficial effects of service-learning on students' personal development may be relevant to work therapy. Thus, Pratt et al. (2003) also speculated that one potential effect of work therapy may be an enhancement in self-efficacy or self-confidence with regard to one's ability to make a contribution to the community through service. Other possible benefits of work therapy may include improvements in social responsibility, empathy, and interpersonal skills (Pratt et al., 2003).

Study 2 was also expected to replicate past research indicating internal consistency and test-retest reliability for the CSSES. Further, based on research demonstrating the efficacy of CBDP (Kazdin, 1995, 1997), a lower level of recidivism was expected for the CBDP group than for the routine-treatment (probation) control (RTPC) group. For the purpose of this study, recidivism was defined as clear and explicit evidence of violating the terms of probation.

Sample and Procedure. Participants included 40 conduct-disordered African-American adolescents between 13 and 17 years of age. Due to felony offenses, these adolescents were on probation in the Montgomery County Juvenile Justice System, Ohio. After matching participants on age, participants were randomly assigned to (a) RTPC or (b) CBDP. Each group consisted of 14 year-olds ($n = 2$), 15 year-olds ($n = 7$), 16 year-olds ($n = 10$) and a 17 year-old ($n = 1$). During a 6-month period, adolescents in RTPC received probation services only. In contrast, adolescents in CBDP not only received routine probation services but also participated in Building Bridges, which is a human renewal program associated with the Montgomery County Juvenile Justice System in Ohio. Adolescents in the Building Bridges program participate in community service (e.g., feeding the homeless, participating in social/recreational programs in nursing homes) for several hours approximately once per week, reflect on the meaning of community service informally with staff members, and participate in recreational activities with peers and staff members for several hours approximately once per week. As part of the program evaluation, staff members administered the CSSES at pre-intervention and at a 6-month evaluation. To administer the CSSES, the participant was lead to a private assessment room and, to control for possible reading difficulties, the participant was asked to respond to audio-taped CSSES items (each statement was read twice).

Results and Discussion. Replicating past research (and other studies reported in this paper), the CSSES had internal consistency at pre-intervention (alpha coefficient = .87) and at the 6-month evaluation (alpha coefficient = .87). With regard to individual item analysis, none of the items detracted from the level of internal consistency (alpha coefficient). Item-total correlations (corrected) ranged from .45 to .83 at pre-intervention and from .42 to .74 at the 6-month evaluation.

For adolescents who did not participate in CBDP ($n = 20$), the test-retest reliability coefficient was high in magnitude and statistically significant ($r = .93$, $p < .01$), replicating findings reported by Reeb et al. (1998). Since it was expected that CBDP may influence CSSES scores, data from participants in the CBDP group were not included in the computation of test-retest reliability.

With regard to recidivism, violation of the terms of probation was observed for 13 cases in the RTPC group during the 6-month period, whereas only 5 participants in the CBDP group violated the terms of probation. This difference in recidivism was statistically significant, χ^2 $(1, 40) = 6.47$, $p < .01$. In general, this finding is consistent with other research showing the benefits of CBDP (Davidson et al., 1990; Kazdin, 1995, 1997). Across RTPC and CBDP groups, adolescents with recidivism ($n = 18$) during the 6-month period had lower CSSES scores than adolescents without recidivism ($n = 22$), and this difference is found in pre-intervention scores ($M = 2.67$, $SD = .56$ vs. $M = 3.43$, $SD = .72$), $t(38) = -3.66$, $p < .001$, and in scores at the 6-month evaluation ($M = 2.80$, $SD = .50$ vs. $M = 3.90$, $SD = .62$), $t(38) = -6.10$, $p < .001$. One may speculate that self-efficacy may play some role in mediating recidivism, but a great deal of systematic research would be needed to examine this possibility.

As hypothesized, the group (RTPC vs. CBDP) by time (pre-intervention vs. 6-month evaluation) interaction on CSSES mean scores was significant, $F(1, 38) = 57.18$, $p < .001$. This pattern of results was fairly consistent across CSSES items; that is, the group by time interaction was significant on 9 out of 10 CSSES items. The main effect for group was not significant, $F(1, 38) = 1.36$, $p < .25$, but the main effect for time was significant, $F(1, 38) = 38.39$, $p < .001$.

Given the significant group by time interaction, follow-up analyses were employed to examine specific group differences. The difference between the RTPC group ($M = 3.15$, $SD = .77$) and the CBDP group ($M = 3.03$, $SD = .75$) was not significant for pre-intervention CSSES mean scores, $t(38) = .50$, $p < 62$, and this finding was consistent across all CSSES items at pre-intervention. In contrast, the difference between the RTPC group ($M = 3.08$, $SD = .70$) and the CBDP group ($M = 3.74$, $SD = .75$) was significant for CSSES at the 6-month evaluation, $t(38) = -2.85$, $p < .007$), and this group difference was found for 6 out of 10 CSSES items.

For the RTPC group (n = 20), the difference between CSSES mean scores at pre-intervention (M = 3.15, SD = .77) and at the 6-month evaluation was not significant, $t(19)$ = 1.11, p < .28. Further, the difference in CSSES scores between pre-intervention and 6-month follow-up was not significant for 9 out of 10 CSSES items, and scores on one CSSES item actually decreased over this time period. For the CBDP group, in contrast, CSSES mean scores decreased significantly from pre-intervention (M = 3.03, SD = .75) to the 6-month evaluation (M = 3.74, SD = .75), $t(19)$ = −8.71, p < .001, and this significant decrease from pre-intervention to the 6-month evaluation was found for 9 out of 10 CSSES items.

In this study, CSSES scores changed in the hypothesized direction in response to an intervention, and this provides further evidence of construct validity. This finding appears inconsistent with results of Reeb and colleagues' (1998) Study 2, in which CSSES scores of college students did not improve over a semester of course-related service-learning; however, as previously noted, the service-learning students in Reeb and colleagues' (1998) Study 2 had very high CSSES scores at pre-semester, perhaps creating a ceiling effect that precluded the detection of self-efficacy improvements. The findings of the present study are consistent with the results of Reeb and colleagues' (1998) Study 3, in which the use of a retrospective version of the CSSES suggested that the course-related service-learning contributed to students' self-efficacy for community service.

Results of this study suggest that the CSSES may be useful in research on adolescents, including underprivileged *at risk* youth with conduct problems. It should be noted that, in general, CSSES scores for these adolescents were much lower than scores observed in Caucasian college students (typically between 6 and 9). It is unclear whether this difference in CSSES scores is due to differences in such variables as age (development), socioeconomic status, race/ethnicity, or psychosocial adjustment. Further research is needed in order to document and understand the differences in CSSES scores across select groups.

Study 3

To some extent, improvements in an individual's self-efficacy for community service (i.e., perceived ability to make contributions through community service) should *generalize* or *transfer* to other domains of functioning. In a discussion of the generalization of self-efficacy beliefs, Bandura (1997, p. 53) writes:

Powerful mastery experiences that provide striking testimony to one's capacity to effect personal changes can also produce a *transformational restructuring of efficacy beliefs* that is manifested across diverse realms of functioning. Such personal triumphs serve as transforming experiences. What generalizes is the belief that one can mobilize whatever effort it takes to succeed in different undertakings.

Further, Bandura (1997) emphasizes that the " . . . development and exercise of capabilities would be severely constricted if there was absolutely no transfer of efficacy beliefs across situations or settings" (p. 50), and he concludes: "Adaptive functioning requires discriminative generalization of perceived self-efficacy" (p. 51).

Some researchers have examined *general self-efficacy* (Chen, Gully, & Eden, 2001; Sherer, Maddux, Mercandante, Prentice-Dunn, Jacobs, & Rogers, 1982). Chen et al. (2001, p. 79) defined this construct as "one's estimate of one's overall ability to perform successfully in a wide variety of achievement situations" or "how confident one is that she or he can perform effectively across different tasks and situations." Chen et al. (2001, p. 63) have suggested that general self-efficacy "emerges over one's life span as one accumulates successes and failures across different task domains."

Therefore, to some extent, an improvement in an individual's community service self-efficacy would be expected to contribute to his or her general self-efficacy. The present study further examines the *nomological network* (Cronbach & Meehl, 1955) of the CSSES by testing the hypothesis that (a) the CSSES will correlate significantly with a measure of general self-efficacy, and (b) the magnitude of the correlation will be in the small ($r = .1$) to medium ($r = .30$) range. In addition, this study attempted to replicate past research demonstrating internal consistency for the CSSES, and it further examined gender differences in CSSES scores.

Sample and Procedure. In a group testing format, the CSSES and the New General Self-Efficacy Scale (NSES; Chen et al., 2001) were administered to 352 undergraduate students (119 males, 233 females) between the ages of 17 and 23 years ($M = 18.67$, $SD = .98$). Participants included 319 (90.6%) European-Americans, 18 (5.1%) African-Americans, 5 (1.4%) Asian Americans, 3 (less than 1%) Hispanic-Americans, 1 (less than 1%) Arab-American, and 6 (1.7%) Other. The NSES, which is an 8-item scale with scores ranging from 1 (*strongly disagree*) to 5 (*strongly agree*), was selected for this study because Chen et al. (2001)

demonstrated that this measure of general self-efficacy has superior psychometric properties relative to the General Self-Efficacy Scale (Sherer et al., 1982) used in past research.

Results and Discussion. Similar to past research, internal consistency for the CSSES was observed (alpha coefficient = .96). With regard to individual item analysis, none of the items detracted from the level of internal consistency (alpha coefficient), and item-total correlations (corrected) ranged from .73 to .87. Likewise, internal consistency for the NGSES was found (alpha coefficient = .88), replicating research by Chen et al. (2001).

Regarding gender differences in CSSES scores, females ($n = 233, M = 7.65, SD = 1.87$) tended to have higher CSSES scores than did males ($n = 119, M = 6.91, SD = 1.99$), $t(350) = 3.42, p < .001$. In contrast, males ($M = 3.97, SD = .63$) tended to score higher on the measure of general self-efficacy (NGSES) than did females ($M = 3.82, SD = .59$), $t(350) = 2.17, p < .03$. Chen et al. (2001) did not report on gender differences in NGSES scores. Using the General Self-Efficacy Scale developed by Sherer et al. (1982), May and Sowa (1994) did not find evidence of gender differences. However, the present finding that males tend to have a higher general self-efficacy than females appears consistent with some research on gender differences in occupational self-efficacy. For instance, Bandura (1997) reviews this area of research and concludes: "Male college students have an equally high sense of efficacy for both traditionally male-dominated and female dominated occupations," but female college students have a " . . . weaker sense of efficacy that they can master the educational requirements and job functions of occupations dominated by males" (p. 432). Bandura (1997) notes that this gender difference is observed even though "the two groups do not differ in their actual verbal and quantitative ability on standardized tests" (p. 432). Results of Studies 1 and 2 of the present paper suggest that community service may be an area in which females have greater self-efficacy than males.

As hypothesized, the correlation between the CSSES and the NGSES was positive and statistically significant ($p < .001$)), and the magnitude of the coefficient ($r = .29$) was in the small to medium range. Each CSSES correlated significantly with the NGSES total score, with the magnitude of the correlation coefficients ranging from .20 ($p < .001$) to .29 ($p < .001$). In sum, the finding that the CSSES correlates moderately with the NGSES provides evidence of convergent validity for the CSSES. More generally, this finding further clarifies the nomological network (Cronbach & Meehl, 1955) for the CSSES and thereby contributes to evidence of construct validity.

GENERAL DISCUSSION

The findings presented in this paper replicate and extend past research (Reeb et al., 1998) and provide further evidence of reliability and validity for the CSSES. First, each of the three studies replicate past research in demonstrating a high level of internal consistency for the CSSES. Second, Study 2 examined test-retest reliability, and the results of this study replicated past research by showing that the CSSES has temporal consistency. Third, Study 1 found that, as hypothesized, the correlation between the CSSES and a commonly-used measure of social desirability was low in magnitude and not statistically significant. Since the items of the CSSES have a high level of face validity, and the CSSES measures an attribute that many would find to be desirable, this source of evidence of discriminant validity for the CSSES is noteworthy. Fourth, Studies 1 and 3 examined gender differences in CSSES scores, and it was found that females tended to obtain higher CSSES scores than did males. This gender difference in CSSES scores was small but statistically significant. Fifth, Study 2 demonstrated construct validity for the CSSES by showing that scores on the instrument changed in the hypothesized direction in response to an intervention. That is, conduct-disordered adolescents in a CBDP showed increases in CSSES scores from pre-intervention to 6-month evaluation, but this change in CSSES scores was not found for conduct-disordered adolescents receiving RTPC. The treatment group also had a significantly lower level of recidivism over the 6-month period, and adolescents with recidivism had lower CSSES scores than did those without recidivism. Study 2 also showed that the CSSES may be a useful measure in studying underprivileged and *at risk* adolescents, including those with problems in psychosocial adjustment. Finally, as hypothesized, Study 3 found that the CSSES correlated moderately with a measure of general self-efficacy, providing further evidence of convergent validity for the CSSES.

The following are some examples of possible avenues for future research on the CSSES (also see Reeb et al., 1998): First, there is a need to more fully define the construct's nomological network by further examining the convergent and discriminant validity of the CSSES. Second, additional studies focusing on criterion-related validity would be helpful in determining the extent to which *known groups* differ on CSSES scores in hypothesized directions. Third, while further studies demonstrating the utility of the CSSES as an outcome variable would be helpful, there is also a need to determine the extent to which changes in community service self-efficacy mediate other favorable changes that occur in an individual's personal development over the course of service provision. Finally, research is needed to determine whether self-efficacy improves with training for community service, and research should ascertain the extent to which the CSSES predicts an individual's effectiveness (e.g., based on supervisor ratings) in the community. As Bandura (1997, p. 525) writes, "The times call for social initiatives that build people's sense of collective efficacy to influence the conditions that shape their lives and those of future generations."

REFERENCES

Anastasi, A., & Urbina, S. (1997). *Psychological testing* (11th ed.). New Jersey: Prentice-Hall.

Bandura, A. (1977). Self-efficacy: Toward a unifying theory of behavioral change. *Psychological Review, 84,* 191-215.

Bandura, A. (1978). The self system in reciprocal determinism. *American Psychologist, 33,* 344-358.

Bandura, A. (1982). Self-efficacy mechanism in human agency. *American Psychologist, 37,* 122-147.

Bandura, A. (1995). *Self-efficacy in changing societies.* Cambridge University Press.

Bandura, A. (1997). *Self-efficacy: The exercise of control.* New York: Freeman.

Bringle, R. G., Phillips, M. A., & Hudson, M. (2004). *The measure of service learning: Research scales to assess student experiences.* Washington, DC: American Psychological Association.

Chen, G., Gully, S. M., & Eden, D. (2001). Validation of a new general self-efficacy scale. *Organizational Research Methods, 4,* 62-83.

Cronbach, L. J., & Meehl, P. E. (1955). Construct validity in psychological tests. *Psychological Bulletin, 52,* 281-302.

Crowne, D. P., & Marlowe, D. (1964). *The approval motive: Studies in evaluation dependence.* New York: Wiley.

Davidson, W. S., Redner, R., Mitchell, C. M., & Amdur, R. (1990). *Alternative treatments for troubled youth.* New York: Plenum.

Kazdin, A. E. (1995). *Conduct disorder in childhood and adolescence* (2nd ed.). Thousand Oaks, CA: Sage.

Kazdin, A. E. (1997). Practitioner review: Psychosocial treatments for conduct disorder in children. *Journal of Child Psychology and Psychiatry, 38,* 161-178.

May, K. M., & Sowa, C. J. (1994). Personality characteristics and family environments of short-term counseling clients. *Journal of College Student Development, 35,* 59-62.

Miller, J. (1997). The impact of service-learning experiences on students' sense of power. *Michigan Journal of Community Service Learning, 4,* 16-21.

Pratt, M., Smith, M., Reigelsperger, R., O'Connor, L. V., Saum, C., Baker, S., & Reeb, R. N. (2003). *Journal of Psychological Practice, 8,* 1-13.

Reeb, R. N., Blumenstiel, B., & Saum, C. (1999). *The Community Service Self-Efficacy Scale: Further evidence of construct validity.* Presented at the seventy-first annual meeting of the Midwestern Psychological Association, Chicago, IL.

Reeb, R. N., Katsuyama, R. M., Sammon, J. A., & Yoder, D. S. (1998). The Community Self-Efficacy Scale: Evidence of reliability, construct validity, and pragmatic utility. *Michigan Journal of Community Service Learning, 5,* 48-57.

Russo, J. R. (1974). Mutually therapeutic interaction between mental patients and delinquents. *Hospital and Community Psychiatry, 25,* 531-533.

Sherer, M., Maddus, J. E., Mercandante, B., Prentice-Dunn, S., Jacobs, B., & Rogers, R. W. (1982). The Self-Efficacy Scale: Construction and validation. *Psychological Reports, 51,* 671.

Community Elder-Care in Tasmania: Examining Whether Caregivers Believe They "Make-A-Difference" in an Urban and Rural Island

Joseph R. Ferrari
Monica Kapoor
Maya J. Bristow
H. Woods Bowman

DePaul University

SUMMARY. Adult caregivers (n = 184; M age = 43.9 years old) working at a non-profit, eldercare program at five geographically diverse sites located in the self-contained, island state of Tasmania, Australia, completed a

Address correspondence to: Joseph R. Ferrari, Department of Psychology, DePaul University, 2219 North Kenmore Avenue, Chicago, IL, 60614 (E-mail: jferrari@depaul.edu).

The authors express much gratitude to Richard Sadek, Peter Patmore, the Board of Trustees, and the staff and volunteers at SCC (Tas). Special thanks is expressed to Garry Askey-Doran, who facilitated this project, assisted in the data collection process, and provided guidance, support, and above all friendship that made this project possible and a pleasure.

This project was funded in part by a DePaul "Competitive Research Council" Award, with ground transportation and supplies by Southern Cross Care, Inc. (Tas), and housing by the University of Tasmania "Visiting Scholar Program" provided to the first author in support of his research leave.

[Haworth co-indexing entry note]: "Community Elder-Care in Tasmania: Examining Whether Caregivers Believe They "Make-A-Difference" in an Urban and Rural Island." Ferrari et al. Co-published simultaneously in *Journal of Prevention & Intervention in the Community* (The Haworth Press, Inc.) Vol. 32, No. 1/2, 2006, pp. 115-131; and: *Community Action Research: Benefits to Community Members and Service Providers* (ed: Roger N. Reeb) The Haworth Press, Inc., 2006, pp. 115-131. Single or multiple copies of this article are available for a fee from The Haworth Document Delivery Service [1-800-HAWORTH, 9:00 a.m. - 5:00 p.m. (EST). E-mail address: docdelivery@haworthpress.com].

set of self-report measures. Results across the five sites indicated that respondents experienced a relatively strong sense of self-efficacy toward making a difference in their local community. However, there were significant differences (controlling for social desirability) when comparing caregivers from rural northern ($n = 45$) with urban southern ($n = 139$) communities, with rural caregivers claiming stronger sense of common mission with others, reciprocal responsibility to help others, and caregiver satisfaction, plus lower disharmony with other members and caregiver stress in helping the elderly than urban caregivers. Implications suggest that community self-efficacy may be high among eldercare staff, but their sense of community and caregiving perceptions may reflect geographic differences, especially in Tasmania. *[Article copies available for a fee from The Haworth Document Delivery Service: 1-800-HAWORTH. E-mail address: <docdelivery@haworthpress.com> Website: <http://www.HaworthPress. com>* © *2006 by The Haworth Press, Inc. All rights reserved.]*

KEYWORDS. Rural vs. urban, community self-efficacy, eldercare, caregivers, Tasmania, Australia

Researchers have compared people living in urban and rural geographic regions, but with mixed results. Keatinge (1988), who compared urban and rural Irish communities in reported rates of adult alcoholism and schizophrenia, found no significant differences between regions. Bultena (1969) examined U.S. urban and rural communities in the Midwest in terms of the number of face-to-face interactions elderly experience with their adult children and siblings. Persons living in urban communities experienced more frequent contact and care from family members. In contrast, Farrell, Koch, and Blank (1996) assessed former state hospital patients now living in urban and rural communities in Virginia and found that persons living in rural communities received better continued care than those from urban centers. Mann (2001) also found significant differences between elderly living in urban and rural communities, with rural dwelling elderly experiencing less depressive symptoms and greater satisfaction from social support than urban dwelling elderly. These studies suggest that a comparison between urban and rural communities on different psych-social variables is a useful analysis because regional differences may emerge depending upon the target behaviors and settings.

In the present study we examined regional differences (e.g., urban vs. rural) in *community self-efficacy* and *psychological sense of community*.

Reeb, Katsuymama, Sammon, and Yoder (1998) describe *community self-efficacy* as the belief that one may make meaningful differences in the lives of persons from their local community. Reeb et al. found that U.S. student volunteers engaged in service learning courses may learn to increase their community self-efficacy through active participation working with local service agencies. Such experiences increase student knowledge of the needs in their community as well as heightened social responsibility to help others (Reeb, Sammon, & Isackson, 1999). We examined whether adult caregivers to the elderly living in different geographic communities outside the U.S. reported differences in community self-efficacy. Because this concept has not been assessed in various settings with adults, no *apriori* expectations were made concerning whether eldercare workers from urban or rural communities would report significant differences in community self-efficacy.

Psychological sense of community focuses on the needs of belonging and attachment people perceive from others (see Fisher, Sonn, & Bishop, 2002). Persons experience a sense of community across varied settings, including different regions of the United States (e.g., Ferrari, Jason, Sasser, Davis, & Olson, 2006) and Australia (Obst, Smith, & Zinkiewicz, 2002). Obst et al., in fact, compared sense of community with 10 urban and 10 rural towns in Queensland, Australia, and found that persons living in rural compared to urban communities reported a stronger sense of reliance on others within their region. Rural community residents depended on one another for safety and security more than urban community residents. We examined the psychological sense of community among caregivers assisting the elderly in Australia living in different regions. We focused on the common mission among caregivers to help others, the sense of reciprocal responsibility to other caregivers (similar to Obst et al., 2002), and the levels of disharmony among members as components of a sense of community as proposed by Bishop, Jason, Ferrari, & Huang (1998). We expected caregivers from rural communities to report a greater sense of community than caregivers from urban settings, because persons in rural regions must rely more on each other given their greater isolation (Obst et al., 2002).

Finally, we examined caregivers working with the elderly in terms of their community self-efficacy and sense of community because this population of health care providers is a rich source of social capital to communities. Because the world's population tends to be "graying," the need for assessments of eldercare workers seems important from social and public health perspectives. In fact, we also examined caregiver satisfaction and stress, two variables considered important to understanding the process of health care management (see Ferrari, Billow, Jason, & Grill, 1997; Ferrari & Jason, 1997; Ferrari, Jason, & Salina, 1995). No examination comparing urban and rural communities on their reported caregiver satisfaction and stress have been reported; therefore, the present study was exploratory without any *apriori* regional hypotheses on these variables.

COMMUNITY-BASED ELDERCARE ON AN ISLAND STATE: TASMANIA, AUSTRALIA

We examined adult health caregivers living and working on the island of Tasmania. This state of Australia may be an ideal site to assess how caregivers living in a self-contained geographic area, such as an island, perceive their abilities to "make-a-difference" in their communities. With a total population of 480,000, Tasmania is the size of the country of Ireland (roughly 198 × 64 miles) with a temperate climate similar to New York State. More than 40% of Tasmania is declared World Heritage Forest Area, and nearly a third of the island state is protected within 14 national parks. Over 200,000 people live in the seaside capital city of Hobart in the southeast section of the island, and around 100,000 others live in the second largest city of Launceston in the north-central section of the island.

It should be noted that several studies have investigated a number of target behaviors among different populations living in the self-contained island of Tasmania. For instance, researchers who focused on the urban capital city of Hobart and its suburbs examined drug and alcohol misuse among community volunteers (Easthope & Lynch, 1992), suicide rates by adult men and women (Koller & Slaghuis, 1978), cognitive and performance skills acquisition with elementary children (Romberg & Collins, 1983), and hotel patronage and drunk driving (McLean, Wood, Montgomery, & Jodie, 1995). Other researchers assessed persons living in either varied southern communities (Sladden & Thomson, 1999: ex-psychiatric patients) or across the entire island (Van Niekerk & Martin, 2001: knowledge of pharmacological management of pain by nurses). We mention these studies because we believe that Tasmanians, who reside in this self-contained island state, have the conveniences of modern, westernized nations yet may be more "isolated" than others given their location. Consequently, Tasmania provides an opportunity to explore how adults offer community-based services to others when it may not be possible to rely on multiple, easily accessible external agencies.

In the present study, we explored adult caregiver characteristics affiliated with an eldercare-nursing program in Tasmania, operated by a branch of the Knights of the Southern Cross (KSC). The mission of KSC is to improve the economic well being and standing of their in local communities by conducting and supporting educational, charitable, religious, and social welfare work. A major charitable activity of the Tasmanian Knights is the operation of *Southern Cross Care, Inc., Tasmania,* referred to as *SCC (Tas)*. SCC (Tas) provides residential accommodations and care/support services for over 800 aged residents in nursing homes, hostels, independent living units, and home care. SCC (Tas) provides elder care services to three levels of residents: *high care residents,* who require constant medical supervision by nursing and health care providers; *low care residents,* who need assisted living, where medical services are not needed constantly but on an "as needed" basis; and *independent living,* where residents live in independent housing units (i.e., "villas") and are provided with medical and health care when necessary but typically not at their house.

The caregivers in the present study included both volunteers and paid employees, termed collectively as "staff." At SCC (Tas), volunteer caregivers did not provide direct health care to patients but offered "quality of life" services (Bowman & Ferrari, 2003). That is, *volunteers* were persons who engaged in contact (frequently or infrequently) with SCC (Tas) residents offering activities, such as reading, talking, sitting, singing, or doing crafts, fund-raising, board leadership, and whose actions may be viewed as enriching the life of residents. *Paid employees* at SCC (Tas) included full-time and part-time employees who were paid by contract or hourly rates and may have health and medical benefits. Together, these individuals provided an assessment of the geographic impact (e.g., north vs. south) of eldercare in a self-contained island, as well as a profile of Tasmanian of eldercare designed to be "in the service of others."

METHOD

Southern Cross Care, Inc. (Tas) Target Facilities

The caregivers in the present study were from one of five primary sites with the highest concentration of residents and employees at the time of data collection (November-December, 2002). Specifically, these sites were:

- *Rosary Gardens*, which is located in New Town/Moonah, Tasmania, a northern suburb of Hobart, on the southeast side of the island. This large site was one of the oldest facilities and included a series of interconnects wings of a one-floor building that went through a series of major physical plant renovations totaling over AU $11 million. Semi-private and single resident rooms were located off corridors with health care stations for staff located in each wing. Rosary Gardens included high care ($n = 184$) and low care ($n = 16$) residents, but no independent living facilities. A total of 71 Staff (58 women, 13 men) participated in this study, a sampling of 36.0% of that site's caregivers.
- *Sandown* is located in South Sandy Bay, a southern suburb of Hobart, in the southeast region of the island. This facility opened in 1998 in a rather exclusive suburb along a rolling hill with 60 low-care residents living in private or semi-private rooms in a two-story building that included an indoor, heated pool, and large conference, lounge, and gathering rooms as well as a free-standing building for small conferences, group meetings, and public gatherings. There also were 34 independent living 'villas' (private semi-attached or attached two or three bedrooms dwellings, each with a one automobile garage, red brick paved walkway and driveway, and lined with flowers. This site has a large kitchen where all meals are prepared for sites located in the southern section of Tasmania. There were 37 Staff (28 women, 9 men) who participated in this study, reflecting 72.5% of the site's caregivers.
- *Guilford Young Grove* also is located in Sandy Bay, in the southeast region of the island. Situated on a rolling hill, this site was essentially one main, two-story building assisting 27 high- and 33 low-care residents living in semi-private or shared, multiple-bedrooms and health care stations located at the center and end wings with several small sitting areas for residents. There also are 38 independent living facilities consisting of private, one-bedroom gray stone villas. A total number of 30 Staff (25 women, 5 men) participated in this study, or 66.7% of the caregivers at this site.
- *Yaraandoo*, which is located in the town of Somerset, in the northwestern region of the island, west of Launceston. Assisting 60 low-care residents in a one-floor building, resident of Yaraandoo lived in either private or semi-private bedrooms along a series of

corridors with no independent living facilities for residents. A total of 11 Staff (7 women, 4 men) participated in this study, reflecting 39.3% of the caregivers at that site.
* *Mt. Esk* is located in St. Leonards, in the northern section of Tasmania, an outer suburb of the city of Launceston. The newest physical plant to be operated by *SCC (Tas)* since July 2002, Mt. Esk was under renovations estimated to be over AU $1 million. A total of 98 low-care and high-care residents lived in semi-private or multiple-shared bedrooms (no independent living villas) located off corridors in a "u-shaped" 2 or 2 1/2 story building. A total of 35 Staff (31 women, 4 men) participated in the present study, reflecting 36.1% of the caregivers from that site.

Participants

There were a total of 184 adults (149 women, 35 men) participating in this study out of a total of 418 potential respondents across sites, for a compliance rate of 44.0%. The mean age of participants was 49.3 years old ($SD = 9.91$). Most participants were European-Americans (93.6%), married (54.4%) or were married (33.4%), with 2-3 children ($M = 2.6$, $SD = 1.01$), at least some high school/college education (64.9%), and living in Tasmania at least 21.6 years ($SD = 5.68$). These participants usually (88.0%) did not personally live at an SCC (Tas) site and most likely (78.8%) did not have a relative living at an SCC (Tas) site. Participants reported worked at SCC (Tas) for an average of 58.39 months ($SD = 20.20$), assisting residents with an average age of 79.32 years old ($SD = 7.50$).

Psychometric Scales

Each participant completed a set of standardized, reliable and valid psychometric measures. These measures included, in random order:
Reeb, Katsuyama, Sammon, and Yoder's (1998) *Community Self-efficacy Scale*, a brief, 10-item, 10-point rating scales (1 = *quite uncertain*; 10 = *certain*) that ascertained whether respondents felt that their service to the elderly provided a degree of empowerment in making important local, civic contributions. Sample items included: "I am confident that, through community service, I can make a difference in my community" and "I am confident that, through community service, I can help in promoting equal opportunities for citizens." The authors reported good internal consistency (alpha = 0.90) and construct validity of

the measure with university students involved with service learning programs (Reeb et al., 1998).

Bishop, Chertok, and Jason's (1997) *Psychological Sense of Community* (PSOC) inventory, a 30-item, 5-point scale (1 = *not true of me*; 5 = *very true of me*) that, assessed a sense of: (a) *mission* (12 items), evaluating the strength of a person's sense of common goals with others in that group (sample items: "There is a clear sense of mission in this group at SCC."; and "There is a sense of common purpose among persons at SCC."); (b) *reciprocal responsibility* (12 items), assessing the person's commitment to offer assistance to others in the group (sample items: "[Staff/Volunteers] can depend on each other at SCC." and; " There is a feeling that persons look out for each other at SCC"; and, (c) *disharmony* (6 items), examining the level of disagreement between members of the group (sample items: "The atmosphere for [staff/volunteers] is somewhat impersonal."; and "Some people feel like outsiders at [staff/volunteer] meetings at SCC." The authors reported good reliability estimates for each of the subscales (alpha $\geq$ 0.70). This measure of PSOC has been used effectively among self-help groups (Bishop et al., 1998) and community volunteers (e.g., Ferrari, Dobis, Kardaras, Michna, Wagner, Sierawski, & Boyer, 1999).

Ferrari, McCown, and Pantano's (1993) *Caregiver Scale*, a 14-item, 7-point scale (1 = *not at all true of me*; 7 = *very true of me*), examined emotional experiences from working as a caregiver for others. Two reliable subscales (alpha *rs* > 0,70) comprised the inventory, including a personal *satisfaction* subscale (7-items: "[Working/Volunteering is adding meaning to my life."; and "Helping [at SCC] is worthwhile to me.) and an emotional *stress* subscale (7-items: "Helping someone as a [employee/volunteer] has burned me out."; and "Working with the elderly as a [employee/volunteer] has exhausted me"). The inventory has been validated with such target samples as health care providers, community volunteers, pastoral caregivers, and persons working with the chronically ill, physically disabled, and elderly (e.g., Ferrari et al., 1993; Ferrari et al., 1997; Ferrari & Jason, 1997; Ferrari et al., 1995).

Reynold's (1982) revised *Marlow-Crowne Social Desirability Scale*, a 13-item, *True-False* measure of social desirability correlated to all the self-report scores used in this study to statistically "control" each person's tendency to provide socially appropriate responses. This uni-dimensional revision of the 33-item Crowne-Marlow (1960) has good internal consistency and temporal stability for a brief measure; high scores reflect a stronger tendency toward social approval.

Demographic and Service Experience Items

All participants were asked to complete a set of *demographic items*, namely: age, gender, educational level, marital status, number of children, length of time living in the community, family history of volunteerism, whether they themselves live at an SCC (Tas) site, and whether they have a relative who lives in an SCC (Tas) site (and what relation that person would be to them, and how long the person has resided at the site).

We also asked each participant a set of items related to their *service experiences*. These included the length of time they worked at SCC (Tas), the number of hours per week they had direct face-to-face contact with residents, number of clients [weekly] they assist, their estimation of the age of their clients, and the percentage of men and of women clients they assist.

Procedures

Data were collected from the Staff through several methods. All participants signed and dated a consent form before participation. Volunteers were mailed to their home a copy of a brief statement explaining the purpose of this project along with a consent form. The statement mentioned that all responses were confidential, anonymous, and used solely for this research project. Also, volunteers were sent the survey items and postage paid, mailing envelopes addressed to the attention of the first author. In addition, through a series of small group meetings with staff, the purpose of the current project was outlined and copies of the statement-cover letter, and survey package distributed along with a postage-paid stamped envelope. To increase compliance, all participants were entered into a raffle (a donated voucher for a dinner for two at a local casino, valued at AU$100) held separate for volunteers and paid employees. Staff had just over five weeks from early November to mid-December, 2002, to return completed surveys.

RESULTS AND DISCUSSION

Initially, we examined whether there were significant differences on the self-reported demographic and service items across sites, by conducting *chi square* analyses for nominal, categorical items, and one-way ANOVAs (with Newman-Keuls, *post hoc* tests, $p < .05$) on interval items. There were no significant differences in terms of age, gender, educational level, marital status, number of children, length of time living in the community, whether respondents lived at an SCC (Tas) site, whether respondents had a relative living at an SCC (Tas) site, length of time (in months) working at SCC (Tas), and the age of residents assisted. However, there were significant differences across sites on whether or not community service was performed by one's parents, χ^2 $(4, n = 179) = 13.46, p < .009$, and presently by one's children, χ^2 $(4, n = 179) = 10.69, p < .03$. As noted from Table 1, participants from Yaraandoo were most likely to report that their parents had engaged in local community service, compared to participants from Rosary Gardens, Sandown, Guilford Young Grove, and Mt. Esk. Also in Table 1,

TABLE 1. Mean Percentage of Participants Whose Parents and Children Have Performed Community Service and Mean Service Experience Scores Across Sites

	SOUTHERN CROSS CARE (TASMANIA) CARE SITES				
	Southern Region			Northern Region	
	Rosary Gardens	Sandown	Guilford Yng. Grove	Yaraandoo	Mt. Esk
	$(n = 71)$	$(n = 37)$	$(n = 30)$	$(n = 11)$	$(n = 35)$
Demographic Items (%):					
Parents Engaged in Community Service:					
	25.7c	52.8b	35.7c	70.0a	48.6b
Children Engaged in Community Service:					
	18.2c	37.1b	40.7b	62.5a	32.4b
Service Items (M):					
Number of Hours per Week in Direct Contact with Residents:					
	9.17b	7.25b	2.14c	22.00a	18.00b
Percentage of Male Residents per Week Directly Served:					
	38.43a	13.68b	22.61b	26.50b	18.00b
Percentage of Female Residents per Week Directly Served:					
	64.00c	86.75a	79.65a	73.50b,c	80.31a

Note. Yng. = Young
Values with different subscribes are significantly different from each other.

Yaraandoo participants compared to participants from the other four sites reported that their children were more likely to engage in local community service.

There also was a significant difference across sites on the number of hours staff spend with residents per week, $F (4, 141) = 3.08, p < .03$. Compared to participants at Sandown, Rosary Gardens, or Mt. Esk, participants at Guilford Young Grove reported they spent the fewest number of hour per week working with residents, while Yaraandoo participants reported spending the most time with SCC (Tas) residents (see Table 1). Participants also differed significantly with the percentage of male residents, $F (4, 141) = 13.62, p < .001$, and percentage of female residents, $F (4, 141) = 9.93, p < .001$, they assisted at their site. Participants from Rosary Gardens claimed they served significantly more male residents than participants from the other four sites, and participants from Guildford Young Grove, Mt. Esk, and Sandown reported they had significant more female residents than participants from Rosary Gardens or Yaraandoo.

The results from demographic and service items indicated that there were many similarities among caregivers who participated in the present study, even though they worked at levels of care, with different clients, in different local communities throughout the island state of Tasmania. It was interesting to note that there were significant differences, however, in the histories of community engagement for respondents across sites, with the caregivers from Yaraandoo, in the northwest section of the island, reporting the greatest history of service. Perhaps, these individuals were more likely to help others in their community because they are in a very rural section of the island where individuals must care for each other and government services are fewer than in more urban sites (Chase-Ziolek & Striepe, 1999; Obst et al., 2002). In fact, participants from Yaraandoo reported they spent the most time caring for residents at SCC (Tas), perhaps reflecting their strong sense of community caregiving (Fisher et al., 2002). Finally, the significant differences between sites in terms of the percentage of men and women residents they serve may just reflect that there are different clients living at different regions of the island.

Assessing Responses to Self-Reported Psychometric Scales Across Eldercare Sites

We then performed a zero-order correlation between self-reported social desirability scores and the other psychometric scores, to ascertain whether there were any tendencies by participants in this study to provide socially appropriate responses to our survey items. Regardless of SCC (Tas) site, social desirability scores was significantly correlated with all subscale scores, except community self-efficacy ($p < .06$). Consequently, we performed a series of MANCOVAs, controlling for social desirability, for each of the self-reported psychometric scale scores comparing across the five SCC (Tas) sites.

There was a significant multivariate effect for site, $F(28, 318) = 1.94$, $p < .004$. Uni-variate analyses indicated that there were significant differences across sites only for each of the three psychological sense of community variables, namely common mission, $F(4, 92) = 4.95$, $p < .001$, reciprocal responsibility, $F(4, 92) = 3.12$, $p < .019$, and feelings of disharmony, $F(4, 92) = 5.05$, $p < .001$. Table 2 presents the mean scores on each of these measures across SCC (Tas) sites. *Post hoc* comparisons indicated that participants at Mt. Esk claimed the strongest level of common mission while participants from Guilford Young Grove stated they felt the weakest level of common mission within their communities. Yaraandoo participants claimed the strongest sense of reciprocal responsibility to help other SCC (Tas) caregivers, while participants from Rosary Gardens, Sandown, and Guilford Young Grove stated they felt the weakest sense. Finally, participants from Guilford Young Grove stated they experienced the highest level of disharmony among caregivers at their site, while Yarandoo and Mt. Esk participants stated they felt the lowest levels of disharmony.

These results on the sense of community indicated participants in our study tended to respond with social desirability tendencies, perhaps in order to "please the experimenter" or to impress their employers. However, when we statistically controlled for those tendencies, we found that participants reported similar rates of self-efficacy from helping others in their community, consistent with studies reported by Reeb et al. (1998; 1999). In fact, as noted in Table 2, participants across sites reported more caregiver satisfaction than stress from their eldercare experiences, which was consistent with research reported by Ferrari et al (1995; 1997; 1999). Nevertheless, there were significant differences in factors related to a sense of community depending upon the SCC (Tas) caregiver site (see Table 2). As was reported by Obst et al. (2002) with other persons from Australia, the present study reported that experiences of a sense of community differed by geographic community. We therefore explored this factor further by comparing rural, northern vs. urban, southern communities served by SCC (Tas).

TABLE 2. Mean Score on Psychometric Scales Across Sites

| | SOUTHERN CROSS CARE (TASMANIA) CARE SITES | | | | |
| | Southern Region | | | Northern Region | |
	Rosary Gardens (*n* = 71)	Sandown (*n* = 37)	Guilford Yng. Grove (*n* = 30)	Yaraandoo (*n* = 11)	Mt. Esk (*n* = 35)
Community	70.12	72.41	64.31	79.64	78.82
self-efficacy	(21.46)	(18.35)	(22.54)	(18.35)	(13.56)
Psychology sense of community:					
–common	36.29**b**	39.48**b**	33.36**a**	42.88**b**	46.10**c**
mission	(8.56)	(8.10)	(9.32)	(10.59)	(15.14)
–reciprocal	38.45**a**	38.71**a**	38.54**a**	45.25**c**	42.06**b**
responsibility	(11.62)	(7.48)	(9.44)	(5.31)	(11.35)
–feelings of	15.91**b**	14.93**b**	16.41**c**	12.00**a**	11.70**a**
disharmony	(6.19)	(4.91)	(6.62)	(5.91)	(4.65)
Caregiver overall emotional reaction:					
–satisfaction	32.28	30.52	29.27	30.29	39.54
	(9.82)	(8.13)	(11.02)	(9.34)	(9.13)
–stress	17.75	19.72	20.28	10.10	14.66
	(9.72)	(9.76)	(8.37)	(4.61)	(8.26)

Note. Value in parenthesis is standard deviation.
    Scores with different subscribes are statistically different.

North vs. South: Comparing Participant Self-Report Scores Based on Opposite Ends of the Island State

We next explored the self-reported psychometric scale scores by caregivers from both northern sites of (i.e., Yaraandoo and Mt. Esk, *n* = 45) with caregivers working at the three northern sites of SCC (Tas) (i.e., Rosary Gardens, Sandown, and Guilford Young Grove, *n* = 138). The purpose of this comparison was to assess how individuals who worked and lived in opposite ends of this self-contained island state might differ in their "sense of contribution" to the local community they serve (Chase-Ziolek & Striepe, 1999; Dixon & Stevick, 1982; Keeling, 2001; Reeb et al., 1998). Because the northern section of the island is more rural than the three southern sites centered around the urban capital of Hobart, we expected caregivers in the north to report a stronger sense of connected with each other and desire to help each other, as reflected in their psychological sense of community (Obst et al., 2002). Because social desirability scores were significantly related to the self-reported psychometric scale scores, we performed a MANCOVA (controlling for social desirability) between participants from the north vs. south on community self-efficacy, psychological sense of community, and caregiver satisfaction and stress, yielding a significant main effect for location, F (7, 84) = 3.24, $p < .004$.

Overall, both northern and southern caregivers at SCC (Tass) reported experiencing relatively strong community self-efficacy ($M = 71.96$, $SD = 19.91$). However, uni-variate analyses indicated that there were significant differences based on geographic location for feeling a sense of common mission with others, F (1, 92) = 12.71, $p < .001$, the desire for offering reciprocal assistance to others at one's site, F (1, 92) = 10.21, $p < .002$, and the levels of disharmony among caregivers at the site, F (1, 92) = 9.06, $p < .003$. Caregivers from northern communities ($M = 45.41$, $SD = 14.21$) compared to caregivers from southern communities ($M = 36.49$, $SD = 8.77$) of SCC (Tas) reported a significantly stronger sense of common mission. Northern caregivers also reported a significantly stronger sense of reciprocal responsibility ($M = 42.70$, $SD = 10.45$) than southern caregivers ($M = 38.54$, $SD = 10.18$). In contrast, southern caregivers claimed significantly stronger levels of disharmony among peers ($M = 15.78$, $SD = 5.97$) than northern caregivers ($M = 11.78$, $SD = 4.92$).

Furthermore, there uni-variate analyses indicated significant caregiver experience scores between northern and southern SCC (Tas) participants in terms of satisfaction, F (1, 92) = 4.43, $p < .038$, and stress, F (1, 92) = 4.02, $p < .048$. Northern caregivers reported a stronger sense of caregiver satisfaction ($M = 38.00$, $SD = 9.70$) than southern caregivers ($M = 31.74$, $SD = 9.67$), while southern caregivers claimed stronger caregiver stress ($M = 18.77$, $SD = 9.47$) than northern caregivers ($M = 13.49$, $SD = 7.71$). These results suggest potential regional differences in persons involved in eldercare services in perceived caregiving experiences, extending the research by Ferrari et al. (1993; 1995; 1997) on this variable.

GENERAL CONCLUSION

In summary, we found that community self-efficacy, the perception that one can make meaningful differences in their local community, was not affected by regional differences among eldercare workers in Tasmania. That is, workers reported high levels of community self-efficacy across different regions of this island state. These results are consistent with past research (i.e., Reeb et al., 1998) demonstrating that U.S. student volunteers, relative to non-volunteers, reported high levels of community self-efficacy. In addition, the present study extends the measurement of community self-efficacy to an international population of adults engaged in service with the elderly.

However, psychological sense of community (reflective of one's need to belong and feel attached to others in a community) and caregiver satisfaction and stress, (perceptions of potential aversiveness in service activities) differed by communities. Eldercare providers from the northern sections of Tasmania reported greater sense of community and caregiver satisfaction than eldercare providers from the southern sections. Although regional differences on sense of community have been reported with other Australian populations (e.g., Obst et al., 2002), there may be alternative explanations for the present results.

In the present study, it is possible the low compliance rate by caregivers in the northern communities (less than 40%) reflected a biased sample of highly motivated individuals. However, we also received a low compliance rate (36%) from caregivers at Rosary Gardens, a southern site for SCC (Tas), making this possible alternative explanation less likely. In terms of caregiver experiences, it is possible that because the northern SCC (Tas) sites did not offer independent living opportunities for residents, the caregivers interacted more with the residents and gained greater pleasure than caregivers at southern SCC (Tas) sites. This alternative is unlikely as well, because Rosary Gardens in the south did not have independent living villas yet caregivers expressed some dissatisfaction from their working experiences. Participants also reported strong tendencies toward social desirability, suggesting a need for social approval in their replies. Even though we controlled for that variable in our analyses, we believe that this tendency among adult caregivers needs further exploration. Clearly, additional research is needed to explore regional differences on these variables across varied communities in general and, perhaps, in Tasmania in particular. Nevertheless, this study does provide some important useful insights into eldercare similarities and differences based on community location.

REFERENCES

Baumeister, R.F., & Leary, M.R. (1995). The need to belong: Desire for interpersonal attachments as a fundamental human motivation. *Psychological Bulletin, 117,* 497-529.

Bishop, P.D., Chertok, F., & Jason, L.A. (1997). Measuring sense of community: Beyond local boundaries. *Journal of Primary Prevention, 18,* 193-212.

Bishop, P.D., Jason, L.A., Ferrari, J.R., & Cheng-Fang, H. (1998). A survival analysis of communal-living, self-help, addiction recovery participants. *American Journal of Community Psychology,* 26, 803–821.

Bowman, H.W., & Ferrari, J.R. (2003). *In the service of others: Functions, management and recruitment of volunteers at Southern Cross Care of Tasmania.* Report presented to the Board of Trustees of Southern Cross Care (Tas).

Bultena, G.L. (1969). Rural-urban differences in the familial interaction of the aged. *Rural Sociology, 34,* 5-15.

Chase-Ziolek, M. & Striepe, J. (1999). A comparison of urban versus rural experiences of nurses volunteering to promote health in churches. *Public Health Nursing, 16,* 270-279.

Clary, E.G., Snyder, M., & Ridge, R. (1992). Volunteers' motivations: A functional strategy for the recruitment, placement, and retention of volunteers. *Non-Profit Management and Leadership,* 2, 349-354.

Clary, E.G., Snyder, M., & Stukas, A. (1996). *Service-learning and psychology: Lessons from the psychology of volunteering motivations.* Unpublished manuscript, College of Saint Catherine and University of Minnesota.

Crowne, D. &., & Marlow, D. (1960). A new scale of social desirability in dependent of psychopathology. *Journal of Consulting Psychology, 24,* 349-354.

Dixon, P.N., & Stevick, R.A. (1982). Urban-rural differences in social interest and altruistic behavior. *Journal of Social Psychology, 118,* 285-286.

Easthope, G., & Lynch, P.P. (1992). Voluntary agencies dealing with drug and alcohol misusers: A comparison of three surveys conducted in London, Scotland, and Tasmania. *International Journal of the Addictions, 27,* 1401-1411.

Farrell, S.P., Koch, J.R., & Blank, M. (1996). Rural and urban differences in continuity of care after state hospital discharge. *Psychiatric Services, 47,* 652-654.

Ferrari, J.R., Billows, W., Jason, L.A., & Grill, G.J. (1997). Matching the needs of the homeless with those of the disabled: Empowerment through caregiving. *Journal of Prevention and Intervention in the Community, 15,* 82-92.

Ferrari, J.R., Dobis, K., Kardaras, E.I., Michna, D.M., Wagner, J.M., Sierawski, S., & Boyer, P. (1999). Community volunteerism among college students and professional psychologists: Does taking them to the streets make-a-difference? *Journal of Prevention and Intervention in the Community, 18,* 35-51.

Ferrari, J.R., & Jason, L.A. (1997). A study of long-term volunteer caregiving to persons with CFS: Perceived stress vs. satisfaction? *Rehabilitation Counseling Bulletin, 40,* 240-249.

Ferrari, J.R., Jason, L.A., & Salina, D. (1995). Pastoral care and AIDS: Assessing the stress and satisfaction from caring for persons with AIDS. *Pastoral Psychology, 44,* 99-110.

Ferrari, J.R., Jason, L.A., Sasser, K.C., Davis, M.I., & Olson, B.D. (2006). Creating a home to promote recovery: The physical environments of Oxford House. *Journal of Prevention & Intervention in the Community*, 31, 27-40..

Ferrari, J.R., McCrown, W., & Pantano, J. (1993). Experiencing satisfaction and stress as an AIDS care provider: "The AIDS Caregiver" Scale. *Evaluation and the Health Professions*, *16*, 295-310.

Fisher, A.T., Sonn, C.C., & Bishop, B.J. (2002). *Psychological sense of community: Research, application, and implications.* New York: Kluwer Academic/Plenum Publications.

Keatinge, C. (1988). Psychiatric admissions for alcoholism, neurosis, and schizophrenia in rural and urban Ireland. *International Journal of Social Psychiatry*, *34*, 58-69.

Keeling, S. (2001). Relative distance: Ageing in New Zealand. *Ageing and Society*, *21*, 605-619.

Koller, K., & Slaghuis, W. (1978). Suicide attempts 1973-1977: Urban Hobart. A further five year follow-up reporting a decline. *Australian and New Zealand Journal of Psychiatry*, *12*, 169-173.

Mann, H.M. (2001). The relationship of physical illness, functional impairment, social support and depressive symptoms in retirement community-dwelling elderly. *Dissertation Abstracts International: Section B: the Sciences and Engineering*. Vol 62, 2492, US.

McLean, S., Wood, L.J., Montgomery, I.M., Davidon, J. (1995). Trends in hotel patronage and drink driving in Hobart, Tasmania. *Drug and Alcohol Review*, *14*, 359-362.

Obst, P., Smith, S.G., & Zinkiewicz, L. (2002). An exploration of sense of community, Part 3: Dimensions and predictors of psychological sense of community in geographic communities. *Journal of Community Psychology*, *30*, 119-133.

Reeb, R.N., Katsuymama, R.M., Sammon, J.A., & Yoder, D.S. (1998). The Community Service Self-efficacy Scale: Evidence of reliability, construct validity, and pragmatic utility. *Michigan Journal of Community Service Learning*, *5*, 48-57.

Reeb, R.N., Sammon, J.A., & Isackson, N.L. (1999). Clinical application of the service-learning model in psychology: Evidence for educational and clinical benefits. *Journal of Prevention & Intervention in the Community*, *18*, 65-82.

Reynolds, W.M. (1982). Development of reliable and valid short forms of the Marlow-Crowne Social Desirability scale. *Journal of Clinical Psychology*, *38*, 119-125.

Romberg, T.A., & Collins, K.E. (1983). Learning to add and subtract: The Sandy Bay Studies. *Wisconsin Center for Education Research: Program Report Rpt No. 83-14*.

Sladden, M.J. & Thomson, A.N. (1999). An evaluation of a surveillance system for patients discharged from the acute psychiatry unit in southern Tasmania. *Australian and New Zealand Journal of Psychiatry*, *33*, 385-391.

Van Niekerk, L.M., & Martin, F. (2001). Tasmanian nurses' knowledge of pain management. *International Journal of Nursing Studies*, *38*, 141-152.

Becoming Better Health Care Providers: Outcomes of a Primary Care Service-Learning Project in Medical School

Cynthia A. Olney
Judith E. Livingston
Stanley I. Fisch
Melissa A. Talamantes

University of Texas Health Science Center

SUMMARY. Medical educators have begun to embrace service-learning as a method for teaching medical students to be more socially re-

Cynthia A. Olney is Evaluation Consultant, Greensboro, NC.

Judith E. Livingston and Stanley I. Fisch are affiliated with the Pediatrics/School of Medicine, University of Texas Health Science Center at San Antonio.

Melissa A. Talamantes, is affiliated with the Family and Community Medicine/ School of Medicine, The University of Texas Health Science Center at San Antonio.

The project team wishes to thank the Regional Academic Health Center faculty and staff, medical students, community-based organizations and their staff, and the communities of the Lower Rio Grande Valley for their participation and support. They also appreciate Marcie Isaacs' help with manuscript preparation.

The Multidisciplinary Primary Care Project is supported, in part, by a grant from the Health Resources and Services Administration, Bureau of Health Professions, Predoctoral Training in Primary Care grant 1 D16 HP 00070-03.

[Haworth co-indexing entry note]: "Becoming Better Health Care Providers: Outcomes of a Primary Care Service-Learning Project in Medical School." Olney et al. Co-published simultaneously in *Journal of Prevention & Intervention in the Community* (The Haworth Press, Inc.) Vol. 32, No. 1/2, 2006, pp. 133-147; and: *Community Action Research: Benefits to Community Members and Service Providers* (ed: Roger N. Reeb) The Haworth Press, Inc., 2006, pp. 133-147. Single or multiple copies of this article are available for a fee from The Haworth Document Delivery Service [1-800-HAWORTH, 9:00 a.m. - 5:00 p.m. (EST). E-mail address: docdelivery@haworthpress. com].

sponsible, patient-oriented practitioners. However, research documenting the learning outcomes of service-learning in medical education is limited. In this paper, written documents generated through evaluation of a mandatory, structured community service-learning experience were analyzed qualitatively to discover the diverse learning outcomes among 24 students who participated in the experience. Preliminary findings indicate that students developed skills and attitudes directly related to competencies of concern in most U.S. medical programs. These preliminary findings may help other programs articulate learning outcomes for their service-learning programs. Further, these preliminary findings may stimulate more systematic research (qualitative and quantitative) in this area. *[Article copies available for a fee from The Haworth Document Delivery Service: 1-800-HAWORTH. E-mail address: <docdelivery@haworthpress. com> Website: <http://www.HaworthPress.com> ©2006 by The Haworth Press, Inc. All rights reserved.]*

KEYWORDS. Community service-learning, medical students, primary care

INTRODUCTION

Medical education has always been service-based. The majority of patients treated in medical school teaching hospitals/clinics are low-income and medically underserved. The challenge, according to Fournier (1999), is to "balance the needs of the patients with the needs of the learners without abuse or exploitation of the former" (p. 258). With rapid medical advances in technology and knowledge, patients become a means to explore and teach cutting edge health care that fit specialists' interests, new knowledge, and available technology (Evans, 1992).

Service-learning is being embraced by medical educators as a teaching method to balance what Evan's (1992) calls this "supply-side" orientation of medicine. The method emphasizes skills and attitudes as well as knowledge, "and thus has the potential to break down social and cultural barriers between patients and health professionals" (Fournier, 1999, p. 258). Service-learning also has emotional outcomes for students, helping them to reconnect with their initial motivation to participate in the activities that drew them to medicine: caring for patients (Eckenfels, 1997). In sum, service-learning may be one tool for reinforcing empathy in medical students and residents and developing patient-responsive physicians.

Training medical students and residents to provide responsive, compassionate and collaborative patient care has become increasingly important to accreditation bodies and opinion leaders within medical education (Federation of State Medical Boards of the United States, Inc. and National Board of Medical Examiners, 2003; Accreditation Council for Graduate Medical Education, 2001; Institute of Medicine, 2003). In fact, the medical class of 2004 will have to pass a clinical skills performance exam with a trained standardized patient to obtain a medical license (United States Medical Licensing Board, 2003).

Involvement of medical students and residents in service-learning may serve another important movement within medicine: community-oriented primary care. Medical students may appreciate better the complexity of patients' lives if they encounter patients outside of the formal medical setting (hospitals and clinics). Some primary care disciplines have begun defining the desired characteristics of community-oriented primary care providers, as they promote a greater community focus for their disciplines (Longlett, Kruse, & Wesley, 2001; American Academy of Pediatrics Committee on Community Health Services, 1999). Characteristics include(a) commitment toward disease prevention in the community, not just for an individual patient; (b) awareness of the many factors (e.g., socio-economic, environmental, familial, spiritual) that affect health care; (c) commitment to using community health resources and collaborating with other professionals to provide access and optimal care to all patients; and (d) advocacy for those whose social or economic conditions or special health needs limit their access to health care.

While the connection between service-learning and emerging priorities within medical education is obvious, the literature documenting its effectiveness as an educational method is limited (Fournier, 1999). Some studies focus on direct benefits to the communities, such as number of patients served through the service-learning curriculum (Christensen, 2002) and improvements to patient care emanating from the assessment of community needs in projects conducted by medical residents (Pierre et al., 2002). Other studies have examined social responsibility development in medical students, measuring outcomes such as increased interest in careers with underserved populations or in primary care (Davidson, 2002), empathy for a specific patient population (Tess et al., 1997), and volunteerism among residents after completing a mandatory service project (O'Toole et al., 1999). Some researchers report the emotional outcomes for the students and residents, like satisfying the early pre-clinical (first and second year) medical students' desire to work with patients (Reittinger & Schwabbauer, 2002).

All of these outcomes derive naturally from the overall objective to develop primary care physicians who are more responsive to their patients and communities. However, the limited range of learning outcomes presented in the literature indicates that outcomes have been determined deductively (i.e., generated from the overall mission of community-based practice). No studies reported a more inductive approach to identifying learning outcomes through the reports and feedback from learners who participated in service-learning activities. Without an inductive research approach, medical educators may not know the depth and breadth of service-learning outcomes for medical students and residents.

In this paper, a qualitative analysis of program evaluation data obtained through a mandatory third-year medical school community service project illustrates the diverse learning outcomes for medical students engaged in service-learning. We investigated two primary questions: (1) What are the learning outcomes described by medical students in their final community service project? (2) How do the students benefit socio-emotionally from the experience? These preliminary findings may stimulate more systematic research (qualitative and quantitative) in this area.

THE PRIMARY CARE COMMUNITY PROJECT IN THE REGIONAL AREA HEALTH CARE CENTER

The Primary Care Community Project was inaugurated in Summer 2002 with 12 new third-year medical students enrolled. These students were among the first 24 full-time students at the Regional Academic Health Center (RAHC), a satellite campus of The University of Texas Health Science Center at San Antonio (UTHSCSA). The RAHC is located in Harlingen, Texas, in the Lower Rio Grande Valley, approximately 200 miles south of San Antonio.

The third year of medical school is a highly experiential year in which students spend a considerable amount of time providing supervised clinical care in hospitals or ambulatory settings, divided into six to 12-week blocks across six medical disciplines. The RAHC students participated in a 24-week pilot program called the Multidisciplinary Primary Care (MPC) clerkship, during which they completed their primary care rotations (family and community medicine, internal medicine, and pediatrics) consecutively. This clerkship was designed and implemented as a longitudinal program across the three rotations, with classroom didactics, community service-learning, and other elements. Of the 24 students, 12 were enrolled in the MPC clerkship from July-December 2002 and the other 12 were enrolled January-June 2003.

The Primary Care Community Project was modeled after the UTHSCSA Department of Family and Community Medicine's community service requirement for students at the San Antonio campus. The primary learning objectives were to develop students' understanding of the role of physicians in the community and the role of community agencies in the spectrum of patient care. The primary learning method was through a structured experience in a community-based organization (CBO) in which students developed a project in conjunction with CBO staff that would address both their personal learning goals and needs of the agency. Because a major goal of the community project was to challenge students to go beyond the familiar roles and routines of the clinical setting, projects did not emphasize clinical care.

Through involvement with physicians and educators in the area, a network of 12 sites was developed. The network of sites is geographically dispersed throughout the Lower Rio Grande Valley. The network addresses needs across the lifespan, and consists of agencies with the desire and ability to collaborate in community service-learning. Sites include the following: a battered women's shelter; senior citizens' nutritional and recreational services center; a birthing center; a school-based clinic with health education outreach programs; a public health department; an organization dedicated to infant and family nutritional needs; agencies serving migrant farm worker families; agencies serving children with developmental delays or disabilities; and agencies serving children with a history of physical and/or sexual abuse. Seven of the sites had prior experience working with health professions students in some capacity.

The CBO executive directors and site coordinators at prospective sites were actively involved with members of the MPC curriculum team in developing project goals and objectives. In recognition of the need to develop long-term teaching partnerships with agencies, the RAHC provided each agency with a one-time stipend to support the service-learning initiative.

Students were permitted to rank-order their preferences among the 12 sites. Their experience consisted of weekly half-day visits over a four-month period. The total time requirement for the community project was 56 hours. The community service project was well monitored.

For instance, students negotiated their service-learning activities with the CBO site coordinators, and students and coordinators worked together to develop service-learning objectives. Those objectives were carefully reviewed by MPC faculty for appropriateness and manageability, and changes were suggested when needed. Project staff monitored activities at each site through phone calls, email correspondence, and site visits.

An evaluation plan was established to assess students' performance as well as the project's effectiveness. Site coordinators evaluated each student's performance, and MPC faculty evaluated each student's oral presentation to peers and 3-page written summary (descriptive and reflective) of the service-learning experience. Evaluation results were incorporated into each student's Family and Community Medicine rotation grade.

Changes had to be made to the project for the second group of students who began the MPC clerkship in January 2003. Some of the changes were based on student feedback collected through process evaluation, but the major impetus came from the Liaison Committee on Medical Education. One accreditation requirement states that student experiences had to be equitable on both campuses. In compliance, the MPC committee re-structured the project to match the one used in Family and Community Medicine rotations at the San Antonio campus. The community project hours requirement was reduced to 24 hours, a time requirement modeled at UTHSCSA and elsewhere (Clark, 1998). Some of evaluation activities were also changed: the written assignment no longer had a page requirement; the site evaluation questionnaire developed for the MPC project was replaced by the one used at the San Antonio campus; and the community project presentation was modified to a debriefing session, conducted by MPC faculty.

METHOD

Service-Learning Participants

Participants were 24 third-year medical students required to complete a Community Service Project. Participants (12 males, 12 females) were between the ages of 23 and 31 (median age of 25) and consisted of 7 Hispanics, 4 Asians, and 11 Caucasians (2 participants did not disclose race/ethnicity).

Data Collection

As explained below, data from the evaluations were used to identify the range of learning and socio-emotional outcomes.

1. *The written experience summaries submitted by students.* These summaries were our primary source for identifying the range of learning experiences engaged in by the students and the learning outcomes they reported. Students' summaries addressed the following issues: project description; project development; project's effect on the agency; measurement of project effects; the most memorable experience; perceptions of the role of practicing physicians in community agencies; likelihood of pursuing future work in community agencies (after medical school); insights during the experience; recommendations to future students regarding the service-learning project; and whether or not to recommend the site to future students (with an explanation).

2. *Site coordinators' evaluations of students.* Site coordinators were given an evaluation form that was to be completed at the end of the community service project, evaluating students' initiative, flexibility, punctuality, rapport with staff and clients, preparation, communication skills, and professionalism. The completed form was presented to the student and signed by the both the coordinator and student before it was submitted to the MPC faculty. Site coordinators were instructed to explain in writing when they evaluated a student as "unsatisfactory" or "honors." Because the ratings were almost universally "honors," there were explanatory paragraphs from coordinators for most students. We analyzed these comments to cross-validate our findings from the students' summaries.

3. *Students' evaluation of their sites.* The 12 students provided written feedback about the strengths and weaknesses of their project through an online questionnaire. We used these ratings and comments to explore challenges to learning discovered in the project.

Coding of Qualitative Data

Qualitative data were coded using guidelines from Glesne (1999). Midway through the first year, the summaries that had been collected to date were read and discussed by three members of the MPC team and a codebook of general themes was developed.

A more comprehensive coding was conducted independently by two members to develop a list of sub-themes within the broader themes identified. The two readers independently developed coding schemes that identified the learning outcomes and socio-emotional outcomes described in the summaries. Reader 1, an MPC committee member responsible for project evaluation, developed a list of outcomes from the codes and forwarded them to Reader 2, an MPC committee member actively responsible for management of the project. Reader 2 compared the codes with her list of outcomes to assess inclusiveness of the codes and to identify discrepancies and additional themes. Themes and outcomes were discussed by the two readers until consensus was reached about the final, inclusive list of learning outcomes. A similar process was used to analyze the site coordinators' written evaluations of students' performance and students' written comments on their site evaluation.

A final cross-validation for the outcomes list was conducted through a reading by other co-authors of this paper. Both were involved in all stages of this project, interacted with students and community site coordinators, read student assignments, and listened to oral presentations or discussions. Final revisions to the outcomes list were made based on their feedback.

RESULTS

Learning Outcomes

Evaluation data indicated that the service project provided many learning outcomes beyond those noted in the literature. The experiences students reported were diverse, although education of patients and health professionals was a common activity. Activities included, but were not limited to, educational presentations for community agency clients and staff, development of ancillary educational materials, literature searches for health information, needs assessments for patient or staff training, development of promotional materials for the agency, health screenings, and labor support (and assistance with natural childbirth). A comprehensive list of outcomes revealed in the students' written summaries follows.

Appreciation of Community Agencies. Many students developed admiration for the agency caregivers. For instance, one student, who worked with midwives at a birthing center, was awed by how the midwives facilitated a birth with recognition of the "dignity, cultural appropriateness and spiritual significance" of the birthing process. Another student wrote, "Community agencies are needed in all aspects. . . . If doctors are to provide the best care possible for their patients, they will most likely rely on some sort of community agency." Another student commented, "It is always such a blessing to work with a group of people dedicated to improving the lives of those who are abused and mistreated in society."

Ability to Articulate the Role of Physicians in the Community. Most students stated that they realized that physicians, to be effective, must know the range of services provided by community agencies to refer their patients. Some students learned that agency staff may be working with outdated information or may be behind in their training and that physicians can assist with staff training. For instance, one student, who helped train personnel providing services related to human immunodeficiency virus (HIV)/acquired immunodeficiency syndrome (AIDS), recommended updated testing procedures. Students also learned that communication is needed between agencies and physicians. Often, these students discovered that clinical rotation faculty members were unaware of services offered in the community. Likewise, they also discovered that some CBO personnel had negative attitudes toward physicians, and some students tried to address this issue through informal education about changes in medicine.

Students articulated the ways in which physicians could support agencies, such as serving on advisory boards or providing financial support for patient education. They also believed that physicians could influence hospital policies in ways that would foster connections between health care settings and community agencies (e.g., hiring social workers, advocating that lactation experts be available in hospitals). One student wrote, "Due to the realities of medical practice, physicians cannot attend to the other non-medical needs that may adversely impact patient health. A social worker can assist the patient to tap into community resources."

Ability to Describe How Socioeconomic Factors Influence Health Care Access and Compliance. Many of the students described examples of how medical care is influenced by social factors. The most poignant account came from a student who traveled with a nutritionist on home visits for clients of an agency dedicated to infant and family nutritional education and support. The student gave an example of two infants with congenital anomalies who were referred to the agency for failure to thrive. In both cases, the student identified socioeconomic factors as a causal factor. One infant, who had a teenage mother and an unstable home life, was apparently not fed the free formula and supplements as needed, until a home health nurse became involved. The second infant had a devoted mother who was poor, lacked transportation to the food stamp office, and was unable to buy food. The student wrote, "My experience with the [agency] home visits has made me much more aware of the plight of these children, as well as the enormous impact socioeconomic factors have on their development."

Development of Patient Education Skills. Most students engaged in some form of patient education. One student was amazed at the level of confusion among community members regarding nutrition as well as community members' interest in his presentation. A second student learned that by educating a group of lay people, the information would be disseminated throughout the community, reaching more people. Students also learned about the challenges of patient education in a society that is so diverse in terms of primary languages, literacy, and age. One student, who presented nutritional information to obese boys, learned that he had to adjust his presentation style for the age of his audience. Another student, who provided a community presentation on asthma, wrote "it was fun trying to simplify the information and take out all of the complicated medical jargon."

Probably the most impressive outcomes, however, were students' development of awareness as to what patient education does for the patients themselves. While a few students commented that they were dedicated to patient education prior to their community service experience, the majority later commented on the importance of education as a key to prevention of health problems. One student, who worked with a reproductive health agency, discovered that patient education can be empowering. He wrote that he was committed to education for caregivers and patients because, "I think, much along the lines of [agency], that education is a part of freedom and freedom a part of rights all humans have inherently." A second student observed the empowering nature of education when working at an agency that teaches parents and families to take care of disabled or developmentally delayed children: "The therapists teach the parent[s] how to help their own children. In doing so, they are encouraging the families to take control of . . . health care and build the critical bond between the child and family."

Development of Admiration for Patients. Some students were moved by the efforts and fortitude of patients. One student working with a child with cerebral palsy remarked on the effort that family put forth in learning about the child's condition and working with her. Another student was moved by her observations of women at the birthing center who delivered without pain medication, labor induction, and other such medical interventions. A third student, participating in a postpartum home visit, was touched by the family who lived in a "shed" who offered a gift of fruit and lotion to the health care team. The student wrote, "It's amazing how grateful these people are who have nothing for themselves in terms of worldly goods but have everything for those that help them."

Experience Using Practice-Related Skills. Many students received practice in skills that would serve them directly in their clinical training: researching health databases; conducting staff in-service trainings; developing training materials, procedural manuals, and policies; providing continuity of care for patients; communicating with patients in Spanish; and working with interpreters. For instance, one student commented, "The interpreter was outstanding and I now feel comfortable working with one. I am sure that this is a skill I will use in the future." One student noted that she observed health conditions that she may not have encountered in a typical clinical setting. Another student was able to practice some basic obstetric-gynecological procedures at the birthing center.

Enhanced Sense of Social Responsibility. A number of students expressed a commitment to volunteer in community agencies. Specifically, they considered providing patient education and services (e.g., administration of vaccinations) in the future. Two other students developed an interest in social issues. One described insights about barriers low-income Hispanic clients face when trying to get basic services: "When it comes to domestic violence, women (and families) are often threatened with the fear of being deported if they access assistance. Victims are often stuck between reporting abuse and losing the sole income provider in the house." Other students expressed interests in human rights issues. One student noted that he recognized that underlying much of the agency's mission is a belief in self-direction and freedom, and he articulated a commitment to this philosophy. Another student mentioned that she had attended a talk on immigration and human rights.

Socio-Emotional Outcomes

Along with the learning outcomes, students described important socio-emotional outcomes of service-learning community experience, as delineated in the following:

Patient Contact. Medical students crave patient contact and the ability to have an effect on their patients' lives (Eckenfels, 1997). A number of the students felt fulfilled by seeing that their projects directly helped people served by the agencies. For instance, several students felt particularly fulfilled by educating clients and addressing their questions. One student wrote, "The most memorable and exciting aspect of my community project was seeing the people of the community actually learn and understand a new topic, and then to walk away with a sense of pride that they now had the knowledge to more effectively deal with asthma."

Social Connection. Some students developed nurturing relationships within the community agency through their service-learning experiences. One student discussed how the elders at her site treated her like "family." Another student talked about making friends with the staff members at her organization: "I love the people who work here and consider most of them very good friends." At one of the sites, students prepared lunch, an expectation of all staff members who rotated this responsibility. One student wrote, "I was quite surprised by how easily I was accepted by all of the women at the center and only wish the members of the medical profession were as accepting of all people."

Learning Outcomes from Community Partners' View

The site coordinators' evaluations of the students generally corroborate the accomplishments and learning experiences reported by students. That is, the ratings were almost universally positive: only three students received ratings lower than "honors" in any category, and usually the lower ratings were for punctuality. Nineteen students received an honors rating for overall performance, one student received a satisfactory rating, and one received an overall unsatisfactory rating because of neglect of duties. This last student was counseled, moved to another site and subsequently received an honors evaluation. Analysis of the site coordinators' comments indicated the following learning outcomes.

Patient Education Skill. Coordinators wrote about students' ability to present difficult information (e.g., breast self-exams, sexuality issues to fathers and sons) in a manner that was non-threatening and to adapt information to different audiences. For example, one coordinator described a student in this way: "He is sensitive to the cultural differences and is patient with the way others express themselves around him." Students also showed dedication to conducting educational presentations, even if only one patient attended. Finally, some community site coordinators noted that students really seemed to understand that health care had to be addressed at the community level.

Ability to Work with a Multidisciplinary Team. The coordinators' written evaluations of students showed that most gave extra time or adapted their schedules to meet the needs of the agency team or community. For example, one coordinator noted: "She has enhanced our team's understanding of the medical role in services to our population." Most students willingly participated in all aspects of a project, including voluntary meal preparation for staff, event planning and scheduling, and home visits in impoverished communities.

Demonstrated Initiative in Improving Provision of Services. A number of coordinators commented that students identified areas of medical information that would help the staff, then made staff-development presentations and created resource materials. For instance, one coordinated noted, "The student readily identified events which posed barriers to women breastfeeding in the hospital and responded with advocacy to change disruptive system and staff practices that deter successful breastfeeding." As another example, a student working in an AIDS outreach organization wanted the agency to adopt a new finger-stick test that provides HIV infection results in 20 minutes. The agency can serve its at-risk individuals better with this test, as many are transient, homeless clients. However, a Clinical Laboratory Improvement Amendment waiver had to be obtained because the Texas Department of Health did not recognize the test; policies and procedures had to be written and approved; and staff had to be trained. The student took the initiative to facilitate all of these activities.

Professionalism. The site coordinators' ratings of students showed they conducted themselves professionally, demonstrating conscientiousness, dedication, punctuality, preparation, and trustworthiness. Coordinators' written comments also indicated that most students were nonjudgmental about clients' circumstances. For example, one coordinator commented, "The student is punctual and I have not had to worry that we are not going to be able to meet a commitment . . . and being able to count on an agreement is very important to our community."

CONCLUSION

This study provides a preliminary demonstration of the broad range of learning outcomes potentially achieved in community service-learning projects designed for medical students. While our project cannot indicate the extent to which each outcome was achieved, it does provide concrete examples of how community service-learning may contribute to the development of community-oriented physicians.

Challenges in implementing this project should be noted. Some minor challenges can be attributed to the students' adjustment to the MPC rotation, while other minor challenges were associated with scheduling or course management issues. However, more serious challenges were associated with concerns that may occur in any mandatory community project involving medical students. These problems required faculty attention and counseling to ensure a good learning experience.

For instance, some students were not comfortable being "graded" by non-physicians. However, the project team felt it was important to emphasize the MPC faculty's respect for the agency coordinators' evaluations so that students would take the project seriously. Other students worried about their inability to communicate with the patient population, which was more than 80% Mexican American, with a large percentage of the population speaking only Spanish. However, some students developed their language skills through the immersion experience and others learned to work with interpreters, so the challenges provided excellent learning opportunities.

Some students were disconcerted about being taken away from the clinic and were not sure how to take initiative in a community-based setting. Again, a key strategy for the team was to stand firm and demonstrate solidarity on the importance of the broader experience and provide support as needed. By the end of the semester, most students saw the value of the non-clinical experience and actually expressed appreciation for the break from the clinical routine.

These preliminary findings could form the foundation of a larger, more summative study on the effects of service-learning on medical students' social responsibility and community orientation. For instance, research could compare residents trained in medical schools that emphasize service-learning to residents from schools with less of service-learning emphasis, allowing a determination of the extent to which the former group demonstrates more of the outcomes noted in this paper.This area of research is important, since medical training programs seek learning methods that contribute to the development of community-oriented physicians who understand the larger context and are able to utilize available resources to improve health care.

REFERENCES

Accreditation Council for Graduate Medical Education. (2001). ACGME Outcome Project. Retrieved October 31, 2003 from *http://www.acgme.org/outcome/comp/compMin.asp*

American Academy of Pediatrics Committee on Community Health Services. (1999). The pediatrician's role in community pediatrics. *Pediatrics, 103*, 1304-1306.

Christensen, R.C. (2002). Resident education in community psychiatry: a model of service-learning [Electronic version]. *Psychiatric Services, 53*, 898.

Clark, C. (1997, October 24). The Patient in the Community: Longitudinal Experience, School of Medicine, University of Utah. Retrieved October 31, 2003 from *http://csf.colorado.edu/sl/syllabi/medicine/clark710.html*

Davidson, R.A. (2002). Community-based education and problem-solving: The Community Health Scholars Program at the University of Florida [Electronic version]. *Teaching and Learning in Medicine, 14*, 178-181.

Eckenfels, E.J. (1997). Contemporary medical students' quest for self-fulfillment through community service. *Academic Medicine, 72*, 1043-1050.

Evans, J.R. (1992). The "Health of the Public" approach to medical education. *Academic Medicine, 67*, 719-723.

Federation of State Medical Boards of the United States, Inc. and National Board of Medical Examiners. (2003). Clinical Skills Exam: Frequently Asked Questions. Retrieved October 31, 2003 from *http://www.usmle.org/news/cse/csefaqs2503.htm*

Fournier, A.M. (1999). Service learning in a homeless clinic [Electronic version]. *Journal of General Internal Medicine, 14*, 258-259.

Glesne, C. (1999). Finding your story: Data analysis. In Becoming Qualitative Researchers (pp. 130-154). New York: Addison Wesley Longman.

Institute of Medicine. (2003). Health professions education: A bridge in quality. Washington, DC: The National Academies Press.

Longlett, S.K., Kruse, J.E., & Wesley, R.M. (2001). Community-oriented primary care: historical perspective [Electronic version]. *Journal of the American Board of Family Practice, 14*, 54-63.

O'Toole, T.P., Hanusa, B.H., Gibbon, J.L., & Boyles, S.H. (1999). Experiences and attitudes of residents and students influence voluntary services with homeless populations [Electronic version]. *Journal of Internal Medicine, 14*, 211-216.

Pierre, C., Lasser, K., Bor, D., Pels, R., & Chomitz, V. (2002). Service-learning projects for medical students and internal medicine residents: The resident's role [Abstract] [Electronic version]. *Journal of General Internal Medicine, 17(S1)*, 87.

Reittinger, T., & Schwabbauer, M. (2002). Creating community-responsive physicians–a service-learning approach [Abstract] [Electronic version]. *Journal of General Internal Medicine, 17(S1)*,100.

Tess, J., Baier, C., Eckenfels, E.J., & Yogev, R. (1997). Medical students act as Big Brothers/Big Sisters to support human immunodeficiency virus-infected children's psychosocial needs [Abstract] [Electronic version]. *Archives of Pediatrics & Adolescent Medicine, 151*, 189-192.

Student Outcomes Associated with Service-Learning in a Culturally Relevant High School Program

Lois A. Yamauchi

University of Hawai'i

Shelley H. Billig
Stephen Meyer
Linda Hofschire

RMC Research Corporation, Denver

SUMMARY. The Hawaiian Studies Program (HSP) integrates the learning of Hawaiian culture with more traditional secondary curriculum in

---

The authors would like to thank the teachers, students, and community members who participated in this study and Jackie Carroll, Andrea Purcell, and Tasha Wyatt for assistance with data collection and analysis. They are also grateful to Barbara DeBaryshe, Ernestine Enomoto, Cecily Ornelles, and Tracy Trevorrow for feedback on earlier drafts and to Sherrice Horimoto and Valerie Dutdut for technical assistance.

This research was supported by the Education Research and Development Program, PR/Award R306A6001, the Center for Research on Education, Diversity & Excellence (CREDE), as administered by the Office of Education Research and Improvement (OERI), National Institute on the Education of At-Risk Students (NIEARS), U.S. Department of Education (USDoE). The contents, findings, and opinions expressed here are those of the author and do not necessarily represent the positions or policies of OERI, NIEARS, or the USDoE.

[Haworth co-indexing entry note]: "Student Outcomes Associated with Service-Learning in a Culturally Relevant High School Program." Yamauchi et al. Co-published simultaneously in *Journal of Prevention & Intervention in the Community* (The Haworth Press, Inc.) Vol. 32, No. 1/2, 2006, pp. 149-164; and: *Community Action Research: Benefits to Community Members and Service Providers* (ed: Roger N. Reeb) The Haworth Press, Inc.. 2006, pp. 149-164. Single or multiple copies of this article are available for a fee from The Haworth Document Delivery Service [1-800-HAWORTH, 9:00 a.m. - 5:00 p.m. (EST). E-mail address: docdelivery@haworthpress. com].

149

science, social studies, and English. Students also participate in weekly community service-learning sessions. Fifty-five HSP students and 29 peers (who were not involved in the program), completed a survey measuring: students' connection to, pride in, and responsibility for their community; civic attitudes; and career knowledge and preparedness. HSP teachers, community members, and students were also interviewed about program outcomes. Compared to other peers, HSP students tended to report feeling more connected to their community and school and to agree that they had career-related skills. Participants believed that service-learning contributed to these outcomes by making connections between school and community life and by exposing students to a variety of careers. *[Article copies available for a fee from The Haworth Document Delivery Service: 1-800- HAWORTH. E-mail address: <docdelivery@haworthpress.com> Website: <http://www.HaworthPress.com> © 2006 by The Haworth Press, Inc. All rights reserved.]*

KEYWORDS. Hawaiian Studies Program (HSP), community service-learning, student outcomes

Service-learning benefits both the community and the participants. It is the latter that distinguishes these activities from community service, as service-learning goes beyond volunteerism in its design to promote participants' learning of academic concepts or skills (Billig, 2000; Honig, Kahne, & McLaughlin, 2001; Wade & Saxe, 1996). For example, students might be involved in organizing a can goods drive at their school. This could be considered service-learning if their teacher integrates the activities with a lesson on poverty and hunger. Many definitions of service-learning also include student reflections on their experiences, student collaboration with community members to plan activities, linkage to curriculum standards, and meeting authentic community needs (Billig, 2000).

There is some evidence that involvement in service-learning improves participants' academic outcomes. For example, Billig and Klute (2002) found that fifth graders in school-based Learn and Serve programs in Michigan scored higher than nonparticipating peers on the state assessment in writing, earth science, historical perspective, and decision-making and inquiry in social studies. Middle and high school students in Philadelphia who participated in service-learning scored higher than matched counterparts who did not participate in service-learning on measures of cognitive complexity (Meyer & Hofshire 2003). A meta-analysis of 38 peer-tutoring studies indicated an advantage of this approach regarding the tutors' own learning and attitudes toward the subject matter compared to alternative instructional methods (Cohen, Kulik, & Kulik, 1982). Other studies indicate positive effects of service-learning in decreasing rates of failure, suspension, and dropping out (Allen, Philliber, & Hoggson, 1990; Melchior, 1999; Supik, 1996).

Service-learning is also associated with higher degrees of school engagement. For example, students in Colorado who participated in service-learning showed stronger cognitive and affective engagement in school than non-participating peers (Klute, 2002). Similar results were shown for Michigan and Philadelphia students (Billig & Klute, 2002).

Honig et al. (2001) suggest that service-learning may yield academic benefits by placing students in contexts where they have access to more varied learning environments, resources, and support. This includes exposure to a greater variety of adult role models and instructors. Research indicates that making connections between academic concepts and familiar information increases the likelihood that new information will be better remembered and understood (Tharp, Estrada, Dalton, & Yamauchi, 2000). Service-learning may assist in making these connections by highlighting the relevance of abstract concepts and skills to life outside of school.

Service-learning may also promote academic outcomes indirectly by promoting personal or social development among participants (Honig et al., 2001). Some research indicates that service-learning increases participants' self-esteem or self-efficacy and reduction in behavior problems (Billig, 2000; Waldstein & Reiher, 2001). These outcomes are then hypothesized to positively affect student learning. Other personal and social outcomes are viewed as more direct objectives of service-learning. One study found that service-learning participation was associated with decreased teen pregnancy, even if the activities were not particularly focused on sex education (Allen et al., 1990). A literature review suggested that high quality service-learning programs enhanced students' personal and social responsibility, sense of educational and social competency, and ability to trust and be trusted by others (Billig, 2000). Further, students who engage in service-learning tend to be more sensitive and more accepting of diversity relative to non-participants (Billig, 2000; Melchior, 1999). Finally, service-learning seems to encourage community activism (Honig et al., 2001). For example, Youniss and Yates (1997) found that students who participated in service-learning in high school were more likely than non-participants to participate in service, vote, and join community organizations as young adults.

THE HAWAIIAN STUDIES PROGRAM

This study examined student outcomes associated with weekly service-learning activities that were part of the Hawaiian Studies Program (HSP) at Wai'anae High School. Located on the western end of the island of O'ahu in the State of Hawai'i, Wai'anae High School is a large rural public school. Like the community it serves and the majority of HSP students, the student population at Wai'anae High School is predominantly Native Hawaiian or part-Hawaiian (Hawai'i State Department of Education, 2002). The school serves many low-income families and special education students, and drop out rates are high relative to other schools in the state (Hawai'i State Department of Education, 2002; Yamauchi & Carroll, 2003).

Founded in 1996, the HSP is a culturally relevant, academic high school program. The program is open to all students in grades 10-12 and integrates the learning of Hawaiian values and culture with more traditional western curriculum in science, social studies, and English. For the 2003-2004 school year, there were approximately 100 students enrolled in the program. During the years in which this study was conducted (2000-2001 and 2002-2003), 3 to 4 teachers were involved. The program involved teaming and looping so that the students stayed with the same teachers and peers throughout their involvement in the program. Throughout the school year, HSP students also enrolled in non-HSP classes.

There is a strong community orientation in the HSP, as the program began as a collaboration between teachers and members of Ka'ala Farm, Inc., a community based organization (CBO) devoted to promoting Hawaiian cultural values. In the 2002-2003 school year, over 12 CBOs participated in the program and were involved in a number of roles, such as assisting in program planning and evaluation or advising teachers on aspects of Hawaiian culture that should be integrated into the curriculum. Community members were also involved in weekly service-learning activities. One full day each week, the HSP students and teachers divided into small fieldwork groups and collaborated on community-based service-learning activities with CBO members.

Students rotated through four different service-learning projects each semester. One group of students worked with professional archaeologists to conduct archaeological maps and excavations documenting the cultural sites and artifacts found in the Wai'anae Valley. With consultation from the governmental agency that manages water use, a second group of students and teachers conducted chemical and visual tests of the area's stream environments. They studied the effects of diverting water from the streams for household consumption. The third rotation involved restoration and reforestation of native plants in the local woodlands and shorelines. In a fourth project, students worked at a local health center, planning and implemented community health initiatives and assisting in patient care.

HSP teachers assigned two students from each project to serve as peer mentors. These students were more advanced and had previous experience with the project. Peer mentors took attendance, assisted students in performing duties, collected and commented on peers' journal reflections about service, and consulted with teachers about students with difficulties.

The HSP service-learning activities were integrated with the students' coursework. For example, in science, students were learning about the scientific method and about concepts such as *ecosystem* and *sustainability*. They discussed how these concepts applied to what they are finding in their stream studies and native plant rotations. In social studies, students learned about the conflicting versions of Hawaiian history and how various archaeological findings support both sides of these debates. The social studies teacher also helped students design and conduct "senior mastery projects," which are individualized activities that reflect students' advanced competencies in the program. The senior mastery project was a HSP graduation requirement, and many students designed these projects as an extension of their service-learning. In English, students read biographical accounts of Hawaiian activists who were involved in activities similar to HSP service-learning projects. In their English class, students also developed their program portfolio, a collection of artifacts and reflections that demonstrated how students were meeting the program objectives. Student portfolios typically included reflections on the service-learning.

This study examined whether service-learning influenced students' (a) connectedness to their local community, (b) civic attitudes, and (c) career development.

METHOD

Student Survey

A student survey, administered at the end of the 2002-2003 school year by an external evaluator, assessed the following constructs: (a) student experiences with HSP curriculum and instruction; (b) student motivation and school engagement; (c) career-related outcomes; (d) civic development and participation outcomes; (f) personal and social development outcomes; and (g) connectedness to cultural heritage and community.

The survey sample consisted of 84 students (55 HSP students and 29 non-HSP students). Among the 55 HSP participants (30 males, 25 females), there were 16 in Grade 10, 20 in Grade 11, and 19 in Grade 12. Their ethnicity included 2 (3.6%) African American, 2 (3.6%) American Indian/Alaskan Native, 27 (49%) Asian/Asian American, 11 (20%) Hispanic/Latino, 41 (74.5%) Pacific Islander, 13 (23.6%) White, and 6 (10.9%) Other. Of the 29 non-HSP participants (10 males, 19 females), 2 were in Grade 10, 25 were in Grade 11, and 2 were in Grade 12. The ethnic background of the non-HSP participants included 1 (3.4%) African American, 3 (10.3%) American Indian/Alaskan Native, 24 (82.8%) Asian/Asian American, 7 (24.1%) Hispanic/Latino, 20 (69%) Pacific Islander, 10 (34.5%) White, and 4 (13.8%) Other. (Since students were asked to choose all applicable ethnic categories, the sums are greater than 100%.)

Individual and Focus Group Interviews

Two sets of interviews were conducted. The first set of interviews was conducted with 3 HSP teachers and 15 community members involved in the HSP in 2000-2001. These 60-90 minute interviews were conducted by a researcher from the Center for Research on Education, Diversity, and Excellence (CREDE) and were part of a larger study on the development of the HSP program. Participants were asked to discuss the initiation and development of the HSP, program outcomes, and future directions. The interviews were audiotaped and transcribed.

A second set of interviews was conducted during the 2001-2002 school year. The external evaluator conducted interviews with school administrators (principal and counselor), 4 HSP teachers, and 9 community members involved in the program. In addition, three student focus groups were conducted, with 19 students in all. Interviews (60-90 minutes in duration) were audiotaped. Interviews probed motivations to participate, activities, outcomes, facilitators and impediments to success, lessons, and ideas for improvement. Focus groups examined students' perceptions of their activities, including likes and dislikes, advantages and disadvantages of participation, and the program's influence on themselves and others.

External evaluators and CREDE researchers analyzed interviews and focus groups using thematic data analysis methods (Ezzy, 2002). Interview and focus group transcripts were examined to identify excerpts related to (a) service-learning in general, (b) students' connectedness to local community, (c) students' civic attitudes, and (d) students' career development. Excerpts were examined to identify patterns in the data across participant groups.

RESULTS AND DISCUSSION

Students' Connectedness to the Community and Civic Attitudes

Survey results showed that HSP service-learning participants, relative to peers who were not in the program, more strongly endorsed statements that they (a) contributed to the community, (b) were valued by community members, (c) were responsible for the welfare of the community, (d) had pride in their community, and (e) took action and made changes in their community (Table 1). On items measuring perceptions related to (a) belonging to the community, (b) understanding issues that influence community well-being, and (c) wanting to take action and make community changes, group differences were not statistically significant but were in the expected direction. Likewise, items measuring civic attitudes, group differences were not significant but were in the expected direction for all but one item (Table 2).

In focus groups, several students articulated why they felt they should care about the community and how service-learning influenced those ideas. For instance, one student described how his teacher explained that they should take care of the environment "because it takes care of us." Another student described how peer mentorship in service-learning helped to perpetuate a sense of community activism by emphasizing the importance of "passing down your knowledge" to the next generations of students. She believed that peer mentorship encouraged students to share information and skills that were useful to the community.

Interview respondents from Ka'ala Farm noted that HSP service-learning builds students' connection to their community. The director of Ka'ala's community learning center explained that the HSP was started with this in mind:

> Our experience is coming from . . . seeing the alienation of our people, our families, from the places that they live. No connection

TABLE 1. Mean Scores on Items Measuring Students' Perceptions of Roles in Their Local Community as a Function of Group

	HSP Students	Non-HSP Students	df
1. You belong to the community.	2.96 (.84)	2.69 (.76)	82
2. You contribute to the community.*	2.89 (.81)	2.45 (.91)	82
3. You are viewed by community members as a valued part of the community.**	2.65 (.87)	2.07 (.75)	81
4. You have a responsibility for the welfare of the community.*	2.69 (.86)	2.24 (.69)	82
5. You have pride in your community.*	3.25 (.75)	2.86 (.79)	82
6. You understand issues that affect the well-being of your community.	3.11 (.69)	3.00 (.66)	82
7. You would like to take action and make changes in your community.	3.15 (.85)	3.14 (.74)	82
8. You take action and make changes in your community.**	2.69 (.94)	1.83 (.81)	82

Note. Responses are on a four-point scale where 1 = not at all and 4 = a lot. There were 55 respondents in the HSP group and 29 respondents in the non-HSP group, except for item #3 where there were 54 respondents in the HSP group and 29 respondents in the non-HSP group. The values in parentheses are standard deviations.
*p < .05. **p < .01.

TABLE 2. Mean Scores on Items Measuring Students' Civic Attitudes as a Function of Group

	HSP Students	Non-HSP Students	df
1. I am willing to take risks for the sake of doing what I think is right.	3.42 (.66)	3.34 (.67)	82
2. I like to help other people.	3.56 (.57)	3.41 (.63)	82
3. I like to help others even if they are not willing to help themselves.	3.04 (.87)	3.10 (.72)	81
4. I am involved in activities that will make people's lives better.	3.11 (.82)	2.90 (.77)	81

Note. Responses are on a four-point scale where 1 = strongly disagree and 4 = strongly agree. For items #1 and #2, there were 55 respondents in the HSP group and 29 respondents in the non-HSP group. For items #3 and #4, there were 54 respondents in the HSP group and 29 respondents in the non-HSP group. The values in parentheses are standard deviations.

to their *ahupua'a* (traditional Hawaiian land division extending from the mountains to the sea). No connection to their . . . environment. . . . That we've been marginalized. A lot of people are living on the edges.

In addition, Ka'ala's executive director suggested that HSP service-learning made connections for students between in- and out-of-school contexts and generally reinforced the relevance of education. The executive director commented, "It goes back to school culture and home culture being integrated. . . . So kids know the value of school."

Implications of these findings are noteworthy. Feeling connected to one's local community is important for high school students, as youth alienation is associated with negative outcomes, including teen pregnancy and drug use (Crase, 1981), suicide attempts (Grossman, Milligan, & Deyo, 1991), and violence (Sylwester, 1999). HSP founders recognized that students at Wai'anae High School were often disengaged from their community and school, and the program was developed to address these problems. In service-learning, students plan and implement projects that are meaningful to community members. This may help youth to realize that their involvement is important and that they can make a difference in the community.

Through service-learning, students may develop positive relationships with community members, extending the circle of adults who serve as role models and mentors. Similar to other rural schools in many parts of the U.S., the teacher turnover at Wai'anae High School is high. Most teachers at the school do not come from the Wai'anae community. In addition, there are relatively few educators of Hawaiian ancestry, as Hawaiians are under-represented in the teaching profession (Benham & Heck, 1998). Thus, service-learning may provide students in Wai'anae with models for how people like themselves can fulfill important community roles.

Career Development

Student surveys indicated differences between HSP students and their nonparticipating peers in career-related knowledge, skills, and motivations. As illustrated in Table 3, HSP students scored higher than nonparticipating peers on items that measured perceived skills in the areas of (a) time management, (b) resume writing, (c) writing letters of inquiry about jobs, (d) working with adults, and (e) leadership. Group differences were in the expected direction but not statistically signifi-

TABLE 3. Mean Scores on Students' Ratings of Their Career-Related Skills as a Function of Group

	HSP Participants	Non-HSP Participants	df
1. I know how to manage my time effectively.**	2.35 (.52)	1.93 (.53)	81
2. I know how to apply for a job.	2.38 (.56)	2.45 (.51)	80
3. I know how to write a resume.**	2.43 (.60)	2.00 (.76)	81
4. I know how to set career goals.	2.48 (.50)	2.34 (.48)	81
5. I know how to write a letter of inquiry about a job.*	1.96 (.64)	1.66 (.67)	81
6. I know how to complete a job application.	2.50 (.54)	2.45 (.57)	81
7. I know how to interview for a job.	2.35 (.71)	2.14 (.74)	81
8. I understand a range of career options that are available.	2.39 (.60)	2.28 (.59)	81
9. I know how to develop a career plan.	2.24 (.61)	1.97 (.63)	81
10. I understand what is required to get into college.	2.44 (.60)	2.48 (.63)	81
11. I know how to work with adults.*	2.70 (.46)	2.45 (.51)	81
12. I know how to work with children.	2.70 (.46)	2.52 (.57)	81
13. I know how to plan a project.	2.50 (.51)	2.31 (.60)	81
14. I have leadership skills.*	2.48 (.54)	2.17 (.66)	79

Note. Responses are on a three-point scale where 1 = not well at all and 3 = very well. There were 55 respondents in the HSP group and 29 respondents in the non-HSP group, except for item #2, where there were 53 respondents in the HSP group and 29 respondents in the non-HSP group, and item #14, where there were 52 respondents in the HSP group and 29 respondents in the non-HSP group. The values in parentheses are standard deviations.
$*p < .05. **p < .01.$

cant for all but one of the other items measuring perceived abilities in career-related skills (see Table 3).

Interview respondents believed that service-learning exposed students to a variety of careers. For instance, a curriculum developer from Ka'ala Farm noted:

They do get to see what opportunities are out there for them. . . . We end up with students who want to be archaeologists. They want to get involved in natural elements [as botanists and environmental scientists]. . . . It's definitely providing a pathway that a lot of them take the opportunity to follow.

Through service-learning projects, students learned details about careers, including the routines involved. For example, a health care professional who worked with students at the local health center indicated that HSP service-learning provided a balanced view of health careers:

What we do is try to give them a realistic perspective [of] . . . the health care professions. . . . Sometimes at their age, they really look more at the glamour . . . what they see as the exciting parts of the roles. And [then they realize] that there's paperwork involved . . . that there is down time.

Students also learned how to prepare for particular careers. An army botanist working with the program indicated that students often asked about her profession:

Some kids who are really excited about the field of conservation have asked us, "Well, what do you have to do in order to get a job like this? Where did you go to school? Did you go to college?"

In addition to enhancing students' career-related knowledge, one teacher suggested that students learned career-related skills:

We send out our students with a better sense of what to expect in the real world after high school. Our students leave with a lot more skills than their peers do. . . . They learn from trained professionals in the different fields, and some of the things they learn, they probably wouldn't get until . . . graduate school.

Another teacher noted that service-learning assisted students in gaining access to various fields. Community members provided information to students about potential job openings and introduced youth to other people in the field. A number of former HSP students were working in archaeology and native plant reforestation, and the teachers thought this was directly related to contacts students made in their service-learning.

HSP service-learning promotes students preparation for jobs in their community. All HSP students prepare a portfolio that includes a resume and often letters of recommendation from community members with whom they have worked. Many of the community members view assisting students in career preparation to be part of their mentorship role. Participation in HSP service-learning presents students with a realistic view of various professions available in their community. Consistent with the missions of Ka'ala Farm and other CBOs involved, service-learning promotes sustainable living in Wai'anae, by highlighting careers that can be practiced within the community.

THEORETICAL AND PRACTICAL IMPLICATIONS

Service-Learning in a Sociocultural Context

The outcomes of this study can be understood from the perspective of sociocultural theory (Vygotsky, 1978; Tharp et al., 2000), which suggests that all higher mental functioning (e.g., beliefs, values, and expectations) originate in social interaction. As children and youth interact with adults and more capable peers, they adopt the language and other symbols of those interactions. In sociocultural terms, they develop *intersubjectivity*–shared perceptions, concepts, expectations, and beliefs. For example, HSP students interact with community members to collaborate on service-learning activities. These interactions may become the basis for shared understandings of community concerns and lead to a collective sense of responsibility for addressing them. Interactions with community members may also help to build students' understanding of potential careers and other roles. As students adopt the same values, expectations, and beliefs of others in their community, they may also begin to identify with community members and to feel a closer association with this broader network.

Service-Learning to Promote Culturally Relevant and Effective Pedagogy

One of the goals of the HSP is to integrate Hawaiian culture into a high school curriculum. Culturally relevant education incorporates the values, goals, or practices of a cultural community to assist students in making smoother transitions from home to school (Osborne, 1996; Tharp et al., 2000; Yamauchi, in press). Research indicates that particular groups within the U.S., such as indigenous Americans, do not perform as well as others on standard measures of academic performance (Kanaiaupuni & Ishibashi, 2003; Reyhner & Eder, 1989). For these students, culturally relevant pedagogy may serve to improve education by building connections between what students are learning in school and what they are already familiar with from their homes and communities. This might involve integrating cultural knowledge into the curriculum as well as using instructional methods that are consistent with interactions that are common to students' homes and community settings.

There are two ways that service-learning promotes cultural relevance in the HSP. First, service-learning is a means of involving community members as educators. Through service-learning projects, students regularly interact with members of the community who are active in the perpetuation of Hawaiian cultural values and activities. Second, service-learning assists teachers in designing more culturally relevant curriculum and instruction. Many of the current and past HSP teachers have not come from the Wai'anae community. In planning for service-learning, teachers and community members discuss what is important to the community and the local activities that might be integrated into the curriculum. Community members serve as models for teachers regarding culturally appropriate ways to interact with youth. Traditional Hawaiian culture emphasizes observation and demonstration of new skills, where the learner is expected to watch silently without questioning the teacher (Pukui, Haertig, & Lee, 1972). Such a method may contrast with a more western instructional style that promotes verbal interaction. HSP educators may choose to adapt their pedagogy to be more culturally compatible or may use that information to better understand students' classroom behavior.

It is also possible that HSP service-learning produces strong student outcomes because it generally provides a context for effective pedagogy. The HSP was selected by CREDE, a national research center, as a demonstration site because it exemplifies enactment of pedagogical principles identified as effective for the education of students from diverse backgrounds (CREDE, 2002; Yamauchi, 2003). In addition, a meta-analysis by the National Research Council (1999) suggested that students learn best and are most likely to transfer their knowledge to novel situations when learners (a) extend their application of knowledge beyond the narrow context in which it was learned, (b) understand the conditions under which learning will be applied, (c) have experience with multiple contexts for which learning can be transferred, and (d) are self-aware of their learning capacities. HSP service-learning provided students with all of these conditions for success.

LIMITATIONS AND FUTURE RESEARCH DIRECTIONS

This study adds to the growing research literature on the positive effects of service-learning on young people's connection to community and career aspirations. However, the findings must be viewed with some caution. Student participation was based on self-selection. Only students who agreed to participate and whose parents also consented in writing were included. Thus, our sample may not be representative of all HSP and other students at the high school. Further, because the number of student participants was small and the type of intervention so specific, the results may not generalize beyond the school. Another limitation of the research was that it compared student responses at one point in time, after HSP participants had experienced at least one year of service-learning. Although the results are consistent with previously cited studies that systematically demonstrate the benefits of service-learning, the extent to which differences between HSP and non-HSP students were due to the effects of the service-learning program or to pre-existing differences between the two groups is inconclusive. It is also not possible to tell whether the results will endure over time.

Future research is needed to continue to investigate the effects of service-learning on HSP students. Such research could investigate whether program components have differential impact on students (e.g., based on student achievement). Research could also address whether participation in this service-learning program influences academic outcomes, such problem solving ability or acquisition of knowledge and skills in science. There is interest, among HSP school and community partners, to determine whether service learning influences students' resilience, school engagement, and valuing of school. Prospective longitudinal research is needed to determine how student outcomes develop over time and whether these outcomes endure after students leave the program. We are interested in studying the interactions between students and community members, as they engage in service-learning activities, to discern whether these relationships mediate student outcomes and if these interactions are more culturally compatible than those typically found between students and their teachers. Finally, research on culturally relevant service-learning in other schools is needed to determine the extent to which student outcomes associated with the HSP generalize to other similar programs.

REFERENCES

Allen, J. P., Philliber, S., & Hoggson, N. (1990). School-based prevention of teen-age pregnancy and school dropout: Process evaluation of the national replication of the Teen Outreach Program. *American Journal of Community Psychology, 18*, 505-524.

Benham, M. K., & Heck, R. H. (1998). *Culture and educational policy in Hawaii: The silencing of native voices.* Mahwah, NJ: Erlbaum.

Billig, S. H. (2000). Research on K–12 school-based service-learning: The evidence builds. *Phi Delta Kappan, 81*(9), 184–189.

Billig, S. H. & Klute, M. M. (2002). *The impact of service-learning on MEAP: A large-scale study of Michigan Learn and Serve grantees.* Denver, CO: RMC Research Corporation.

Cohen, P. A., Kulik, J. A., & Kulik, C. C. (1982). Educational outcomes of tutoring: A meta-analysis of findings. *American Educational Research Journal, 19*, 237-248.

Crase, D. (1981). Declining health behavior of adolescents: A measure of alienation. *High School Journal, 64*(5), 213-216.

CREDE (2002). *The five standards for effective pedagogy.* Retrieved December 19, 2003, from University of California, Center for Research on Education, Diversity, and Excellence Web site: http://www.crede.ucsc.edu/standards/standards.html

Ezzy, D. (2002). *Qualitative analysis: Practice and innovations.* New York: Routledge.

Grossman, D. C., Milligan, B. C., & Deyo, R. A. (1991). Risk Factors for suicide attempts among Navajo adolescents. *American Journal of Public Health, 81*(7), 870-874.

Hawai'i State Department of Education (2002). *Wai'anae High School school status and improvement report, Fall 2002.* Retrieved July 31, 2003 from the Hawai'i State Department of Education Web site: http://www.arch.k12.hi.us/school/ssir/2002/leeward.html

Honig, M. I. Kahne, J., McLaughlin, M. W. (2001). School-community connections: Strengthening opportunity to learn and opportunity to teach. In V. Richardson (Ed.), *Handbook of research on teaching* (4th ed.), pp. 998-1028.

Kanaiaupuni, S. M., & Ishibashi, K. (2003, June). *Left behind? The status of Hawaiian students in Hawai'i public schools.* (PASE Report No. 02.03.13). Honolulu, HI: Kamehameha Schools.

Klute, M. M. (2002) *Evaluation of the Colorado Learn and Serve Program.* Denver, CO: RMC Research Corporation.

Melchior, A. (1999). *Summary report: National evaluation of Learn and Serve America.* Waltham, MA: Center for Human Resources, Brandeis University.

Meyer, S., & Hofshire, L. (2003). *Evaluation of the Michigan Learn and Serve Program.* Denver, CO: RMC Research Corporation.

National Research Council (1999). *How people learn: Brain, mind, experience, and school.* Washington, DC: National Academy Press.

Osborne, A. B. (1996). Practice into theory into practice: Culturally relevant pedagogy for students we have marginalized and normalized. *Anthropology and Education Quarterly, 27*, 285-314.

Pukui, M. K., Haertig, E. W., & Lee, C. A. (1972). *Nānā i ke kumu (Look to the source).* Honolulu, HI: Hui Hānai.

Reyhner, J., & Eder, J., (1989). *A history of Indian education.* Billings, MT: Eastern Montana College.

Supik, J. (1996). *Valued youth partnerships: Programs in caring.* San Antonio, TX: Intercultural Research and Development Association.

Sylwester, R. (1999). In search of the roots of adolescent aggression. *Educational Leadership, 57*(1), 65-69.

Tharp, R. G., Estrada, P., Dalton, S., & Yamauchi, L. A. (2000). *Teaching transformed: Achieving excellence, fairness, inclusion, and harmony.* Boulder, CO: Westview.

Vygotsky, L. S. (1978). *Mind in society: The development of higher psychological processes* (M. Cole, V. John-Steiner, S. Scribner & E. Souberman, Eds. & Trans.). Cambridge, MA: Harvard University Press.

Wade, R. C., & Saxe, D. W. (1996). Community service-learning in the social studies: Historical roots, empirical evidence, critical issues. *Theory and Research in Social Education, 24,* 331-359.

Waldstein, F. A., & Reiher, T. C. (2001). Service-learning and students' personal and civic development. *Journal of Experiential Education, 24,* 7-13.

Yamauchi, L. A. (in press). Culture matters: Research and development of culturally relevant instruction. In C. R. O'Donnell & L. A. Yamauchi (Eds.), *Culture and context in human behavior change: Theory, research, and applications.* New York: Peter Lang.

Yamauchi, L. A. (2003). Making school relevant for at-risk students: The Waiʻanae High School Hawaiian Studies Program. *Journal of Education for Students Placed at Risk, 8,* 379-390.

Yamauchi, L. A., & Carroll, J. H. (2003, September). *Fostering Hawaiian youth wellness through community involvement in a high school program.* Paper presented at the Kamehameha Schools Research Conference on the Education and Well-Being of Hawaiians, Kahuku, HI.

Youniss, J., & Yates, M. (1997). *Community service and social responsibility in youth.* Chicago: University of Chicago Press.

Index

Page numbers followed by the letter "t" designate tables.

BOOK ORDER FORM!

Order a copy of this book with this form or online at:
http://www.HaworthPress.com/store/product.asp?sku= 5684

Community Action Research:
Benefits to Community Members and Service Providers

____ in softbound at $22.95 ISBN-13: 978-0-7890-3047-4 / ISBN-10: 0-7890-3047-0.
____ in hardbound at $39.95 ISBN-13: 978-0-7890-3046-7 / ISBN-10: 0-7890-3046-2.

COST OF BOOKS _____

POSTAGE & HANDLING _____
US: $4.00 for first book & $1.50
for each additional book
Outside US: $5.00 for first book
& $2.00 for each additional book.

SUBTOTAL _____

In Canada: add 7% GST. _____

STATE TAX _____
CA, IL, IN, MN, NJ, NY, OH, PA & SD residents
please add appropriate local sales tax.

FINAL TOTAL _____

If paying in Canadian funds, convert
using the current exchange rate,
UNESCO coupons welcome.

❑ **BILL ME LATER:**
Bill-me option is good on US/Canada/
Mexico orders only; not good to jobbers,
wholesalers, or subscription agencies.

❑ **Signature** _____

❑ **Payment Enclosed: $**_____

❑ **PLEASE CHARGE TO MY CREDIT CARD:**
❑ Visa ❑ MasterCard ❑ AmEx ❑ Discover
❑ Diner's Club ❑ Eurocard ❑ JCB

Account #_____

Exp Date_____

Signature_____
(Prices in US dollars and subject to change without notice.)

PLEASE PRINT ALL INFORMATION OR ATTACH YOUR BUSINESS CARD

Name

Address

City   State/Province   Zip/Postal Code

Country

Tel   Fax

E-Mail

May we use your e-mail address for confirmations and other types of information? ❑Yes ❑No We appreciate receiving
your e-mail address. Haworth would like to e-mail special discount offers to you, as a preferred customer.
We will never share, rent, or exchange your e-mail address. We regard such actions as an invasion of your privacy.

Order from your **local bookstore** or directly from
The Haworth Press, Inc. 10 Alice Street, Binghamton, New York 13904-1580 • USA
Call our toll-free number (1-800-429-6784) / Outside US/Canada: (607) 722-5857
Fax: 1-800-895-0582 / Outside US/Canada: (607) 771-0012
E-mail your order to us: orders@HaworthPress.com

For orders outside US and Canada, you may wish to order through your local
sales representative, distributor, or bookseller.
For information, see http://HaworthPress.com/distributors

(Discounts are available for individual orders in US and Canada only, not booksellers/distributors.)

Please photocopy this form for your personal use.
www.HaworthPress.com

BOF06